Creative Eng in Palliative Care

New perspectives on user involveme.

Edited by

LUCINDA JARRETT

Artistic Director
Rosetta Life

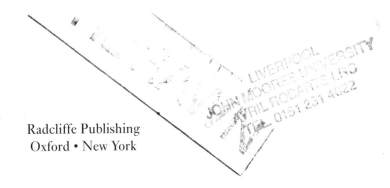

Radcliffe Publishing
Oxford • New York

Radcliffe Publishing Ltd
18 Marcham Road
Abingdon
Oxon OX14 1AA
United Kingdom

www.radcliffe-oxford.com
Electronic catalogue and worldwide online ordering facility

British Library Cataloguing in Publication Data

A catalogue record for this book is available from the British Library.

ISBN-13: 978 1 84619 158 9

Typeset by Phoenix Photosetting, Chatham, Kent
Printed and bound by TJI Digital, Padstow, Cornwall

Contents

*Paula Clarke's contribution to this book is included as a result of her wishes prior to her death and of her partner's recent agreement.

Dedicated to Paul Laking

And the many palliative care service users I have met over the past ten years who have showed me how to live a better life.

Thanks to all those who have contributed to the development of user involvement in palliative care, and in particular to Michele Angelo Petrone.

Foreword

How things began

Once upon a time, there was a very clear idea of what should happen if someone had a problem, or they were ill and wanted some kind of help. Because governments had been made to realise that life could be very hard for people if they didn't have much money, the state in Britain had set up its own services that anyone could use. This included schools and housing; money if you were sick, pensions, help with children and so on. But people were most proud of and talked most about the health services that the government set up. The idea was that everyone should have the best healthcare available and it would be free 'at the point of delivery'. Of course, even before that, for a very long time, people in great need could get help from churches and charities, although there wasn't always enough to go round. Also if you had lots of money, you could go and buy what you wanted and wouldn't have to go anywhere near officials.

However, as people began to get used to the services provided by the government and forgot what it had been like before, they began to think more carefully about what they were like. They realised that although they were often very good services, they weren't always quite what they wanted (especially if they came from minority communities), it was sometimes difficult and took a long time to get them and the quality was not always quite the best. They also noticed other things. They noticed that people who worked in these services, even when they were excellent, sometimes didn't seem to realise how important it could feel to be treated as though you had a mind of your own and that you might have opinions and views of your own. You wanted to know things and play an active part in what happened to you.

Wanting to make a difference

People talked about feeling that health services could put you in a passive position. They talked about 'paternalistic' services; that is services which were there to do 'good for you', but didn't really involve you actively in the process.

And then people started to talk about *getting involved*. They began to wonder if services, like health and care services, really could be the best, if patients and service users didn't have any say or control over them. 'They say they know best, but I know myself better than they can'. 'Ok they have been trained and read the books, but what I know, I know from direct experience. That is important too.'

This book is about user involvement. It is concerned with sharing knowledge and experience about user involvement in palliative care and making it more real for the future. But two other issues are central to it. First, is its commitment to an imaginative approach to user involvement. Second, is the way that it highlights that while people who use palliative care services face particular difficulties and barriers, this is no reason why they cannot be involved if they wish to. Some commentators have highlighted the ethical and practical problems around involving palliative care service users. People may have limited time. They may well be very ill, tired and facing discomfort. All these issues are true, but they should never be advanced as reasons why people who want to cannot be involved. They are also a key reason why imaginative and supportive approaches to user involvement, which this book highlights, are so important here.

There is one more issue to remember. In modern times, the importance of 'end of life care' was highlighted by the pioneers of the voluntary hospice movement. They emphasised the importance of palliative care being based on an holistic approach that took account of all aspects of people's lives and deaths; medical, social, spiritual and material. More recently the work of the independent hospice movement has been complemented by the development and expansion of specialist palliative care in state provision. This is another reason why it is now so important to take forward user involvement energetically, so that regardless of which sector people receive support from, they can expect equal opportunities in terms of their views and voices being listened to.

It is helpful to be clearer about what user involvement can mean. It is a complex idea and there is little agreement about its meaning. It can mean many things. It can be a process, a value, a means and an end. It can have very formal and structured expressions. It can also be something that we do so routinely, that we don't even realise we are doing it!

We wrote an initial statement about user involvement for this book to help contributors and we are incorporating it here. But there are no absolutes in this field. As you will see a little later, the one thing that people most associate with 'good' user involvement is that it leads to positive change in line with what they want. That is a light we should never lose sight of, but much else about user involvement is still the subject of lively discussion.

What is user involvement?

It is not an easy exercise to define user involvement. Other terms are also used as well, like patient and public involvement, consumer and citizen involvement and participation. There is no agreement about what service user involvement or these other terms mean.

However, there are some common themes which seem to be associated with user involvement.

User involvement is about more than filling in 'satisfaction' surveys/questionnaires. It is not just about being a passive 'data source'. It is a more active process, involving people in speaking for and acting for themselves. It is associated with other terms like empowerment and partnership.

People can be involved in all sorts of ways. User involvement often means being consulted or being asked to be members of formal groups and bodies with a focus on user involvement. Some people feel that 'consultation' doesn't really count as user involvement, because it can be so limited. People worry about 'tokenism'.

User involvement however can mean much more. This includes receiving a budget which you control; active consultation (where there is a commitment to listen to your views) It can mean being able to contribute your experience, ideas and views in all sorts of ways. It can take many different expressions. It need not be based on conventional meetings and letter writing. All sorts of ideas have been developed, from having a party to work out what you want to do, creating poster displays, organising meet and greet sessions, to running your own workshop or event.

It can be something that people do as individuals and as groups. User involvement can take all kinds of forms, from people getting together to set up their own independent 'user controlled' organisations' (seen by many service users as the most important expression of user involvement), to one off events, conferences (which they run), gatherings, performance, poetry, arts, cultural activities. User involvement can be fun, as well as a serious business. What defines it is that the purpose is for people to have opportunities to speak for themselves and for their perspectives to be respected and acted on. Good user involvement respects difference, addresses diversity and seeks to be as inclusive as possible. This means, for example, ensuring that people can take part if they have physical or sensory impairments, learning difficulties, experience of mental distress or do not communicate verbally or speak English, or where English is not their first language.

The most valued kinds of user involvement are where involvement leads to change in line with service users' rights and needs; where people are directly involved in decision making and have some financial control. In a nutshell good user involvement is involvement which makes a difference and can lead to discernible change and improvement in people's lives. It is about enabling service users to be involved as part of a process of development and change in line with what they would like to see, recognising that different interests also have to be negotiated.

User involvement can be related to all sorts of activities, including training professionals, planning and managing services, inspection and service monitoring, defining quality standards, research and evaluation, producing learning materials, staff recruitment and promotion and in shaping, developing and assessing workers' practice.

User involvement activities can include support and mutual aid dimensions as well as being concerned with sharing views and making change. These two dimensions can often be blurred and overlap as service users seek to gain confidence and capacity to participate on more equal terms.

All these issues crop up in this book. This book brings together a wide range of exciting experiences in this field. It shows just how much has been achieved in a very short time. In our view, user involvement has come relatively late to palliative care, perhaps because of the anxieties professionals have had about the capacity of service users to be involved without damaging personal cost. This is time for celebration of achievements so far. But there is still a long way to go and hopefully this book and its contributions will help many more in palliative care, both practitioners and service users to take forward this life enhancing enterprise.

A participatory process

There is one last point that needs to be made here. This book has itself had to address issues of user involvement in its own development. Its production has been a participatory process. People with many different backgrounds and experience have contributed to it. It includes accounts from a range of different perspectives. Some of the people whose contributions are offered here are not used to writing and certainly don't have experience of writing professionally. For some people English is not their first language.

One of the aims in producing this book has been to make it possible for people to contribute their ideas and perspectives regardless of conventional familiarity and expertise with writing. The aim has been to offer support wherever necessary to enable people to offer their unique perspectives and accounts of their experience.

This means that there are many different perspectives in this book and they are offered as people have wanted to offer them. Contributions have been put together in different ways and while the aim has been to produce an accessible and readable book, no attempt has been made to homogenise people's styles or to impose one standard narrative on them. This would defeat the object of the book, contradict its commitment to participation and ignore the complex ethical and philosophical issues involved.

Instead the goal has been to respect the process of producing people's contribution as they prefer, trying to be transparent about how this was achieved. Where people have been supported to make their voices heard, this involvement has not been denied, but equally supporters have not put themselves or their views into the picture unnecessarily. The aim has been to enable people to be able to 'do it their way' with a real sense of control and to be able to communicate their unique words, voices and experience. This is and will always be a key potential of user involvement.

Suzy Croft and Peter Beresford
August 2007

Peter Beresford OBE is Professor of Social Policy and Director of the Centre for Citizen Participation at Brunel University. He is also Chair of Shaping Our Lives: the national user network. Shaping Our Lives is an independent user controlled organisation which is funded by the Department of Health to increase user involvement at local and national levels in health and social care and raise the standard of services and support service users receive. Peter Beresford is also a Visiting Fellow at the School of Social Work and Psycho-social Studies at the University of East Anglia. He is a long-term user of mental health services and active in the mental health service users/survivors movement. He is also a Trustee of the Social Care Institute for Excellence.

Suzy Croft is a senior social worker at St John's Palliative Care Centre and Research Fellow at the Centre for Citizen Participation at Brunel University. She is a trustee of two leading UK palliative care organisations and she is a member of the editorial collective of *Critical Social Policy*.

Preface

In 1996 I set up a project called Life Stories. The aim of this was to enable people to find ways to tell stories. I had been working at the BBC for three years in science documentary production where I loved meeting people and encouraging them to tell their stories but found it hard to reconcile the intensity and conviction of each individual story with the need to make it fit into a science narrative that was owned by a director/producer and copyrighted by the production house. I wanted to find a place to work where people could own the stories they told.

I began working with a movement therapist, Filipa Pereira Stubbs and we spent several months exploring ways of using movement to enable people to find ways of accessing the stories that were important to them and their families. When we approached hospices with the idea of enabling people using their service to tell their own stories for themselves, the idea was much welcomed. 'The user's voice' was at the heart of our approach and this was immediately recognised by palliative care services. The voice of the service user has always been significant in healthcare. The celebration of that voice is particularly significant for the most vulnerable and frail service users, people who are living with life threatening and long-term illnesses. For many patients, chronic illness means long-term dependence on disability benefits and the process of qualifying for this can be demoralising and psychologically debilitating. For patients who are facing death, the process of disappearing from a cultural arena is one of increasing powerlessness. Finding voice enables people to choose whether to regain a role in their social and cultural arena. This choice begins with the active engagement in communication between patient and family and between patient and healthcare providers.

A London hospice user who could not communicate her despair welcomed the chance to write a poem that contained it and communicated it directly to her social workers or counsellors. Her emotions were held by the form of the poem and the form itself gives clarity to complex emotions. A mother with young children who worried that her voice would be lost as her children grew up without her welcomed the chance to make a video that left a lasting legacy of her daily life with her family through her illness. She was able to offer her children her voice when she worried that they would be left with nothing.

The creative arts clearly have a large role to play in enabling people to find a shape to hold their individual stories. This personal creativity also has a public and political role in enabling people to choose whether or not to get more involved in the places where they receive care. The arts make an effective public statement. If a person is able to display their artwork on a hospice/hospital wall it enables him/her to hold some ownership of that space. The artist becomes a stakeholder in the institution because their artwork is displayed. Similarly a performance/film screening/poetry reading enables someone to take ownership of an event in the place where they receive their care and in so doing feel more responsible for what takes place in that space.

At a personal level, families who may feel that they cannot cope with the management of the disease that is overtaking the person they love may manage to take control of their daily lives by becoming involved in a creative project. Sorting out the photos, editing a manuscript, viewing rough cuts of a film quickly becomes a family process and in this way carers are more able to get more involved in aspects of the management of the lives of those who are seriously ill.

Some individuals may want to get involved in public campaigning and in addressing the issues that face people who are living with serious illnesses. Maxine Edgington worked with Billy Bragg and Rosetta Life to create a song entitled 'We Laughed'. This was released as a single into the UK Charts and reached Number 11 in October 2005. Maxine welcomed the chance to speak about palliative care, the issues facing single mothers living with illnesses and embraced the opportunity to challenge the stereotype of the passive victim of suffering, replacing this with the positive image of a celebratory love song. She became involved in changing the representation of the dying. Others choose to become involved in education and the delivery of medical care. Groups have been set up to enable patients to talk to doctors and explore with them specific training issues – communication, understanding pain, addressing emotions, for example.

The links between finding voice and becoming involved in the delivery of care are not necessarily direct, but there are clear paths between them. An artist activist like Michele Angelo Petrone who has made a lifetime's commitment to placing the emotions of the patient at the forefront of the agenda of doctor-patient communications has chosen to make his art a statement of soul pain and has made public the need to making soul pain present in healthcare institutions by curating exhibitions in hospitals and hospices across the country. However, most people living with a life threatening illness are concerned to keep themselves and their families as stable and safe as possible and use their art to restore their self-esteem on a personal level.

The process of finding voice is significant in giving people the confidence to express themselves to family, healthcare workers, friends and colleagues. It can be quite distinct from 'user involvement'. However, if a politicised and active collective users voice is to make a significant contribution towards the delivery of healthcare, it could be the first step towards enabling people to take choices about how they want to become involved. As Suzy Croft and Peter Beresford argue in the foreword, 'user involvement' may mean many different things. It does not necessarily mean attending users forums or filling in questionnaires about the delivery of care in a day centre.

This book outlines the role that the arts can play in enabling people to make choices about how they would like to take ownership of their identity, their lives they lead with illness and the places where they receive care. *Creative Engagement in Palliative Care: new perspectives on user involvement* invites us to be bold and imaginative about how we take forward ideas about user involvement and how we not only build on the successes of the past but also offer new ways forward for the future of people living with life threatening illnesses.

This book sets out to explore how people can find their voice; it looks at some of the opportunities available for people to use their voice through examples that others have offered; it looks at the links between personal creativity and public identity and the role the arts, public education and medical education play in delivering change. It is clear that art is transformational. The role of metaphor – which often lies at the heart of art – is to show things in another way, to transform our seeing of objects, experience, the world. In the context of life threatening illnesses, the arts enable people to find their voice to express their identity and to encourage a wider audience to see people differently.

The book is divided into four parts, Finding a voice, Developing support, Advancing involvement and Models of good practice that offer practical guides for people who would like to implement some ideas into their own practice. The first part is dedicated to the development of individual narratives. Chapter 2 contains the narratives of three people who were all at St Lukes Hospice in Basildon in 2003: an artist, a service user and a doctor. The three people demonstrate the different languages we negotiate when trying to find our voice – the medical narrative of care, the creative language of cultural debate and the personal voice of each individual. Some of the narratives are the isolated voices of strong service users. A single patient may choose to develop their work and with increased confidence make a powerful statement, as Katherine Vaughan-Williams made with her work, 'A Guide to Living with Cancer According to PG Wodehouse', reprinted here in full in Chapter 3. This was a text that was developed in the hospice and performed in public at Hampstead Theatre, July 2003. In making a public statement she was able to make clear her own reflections about living with cancer.

Maxine Edgington's song celebrated her love for her daughter. Maxine wanted to make a public statement about love of a mother for her daughter and after the song had been produced wanted to celebrate the impact of the song on her life. Her song made a clear statement about the ability of people facing death to celebrate life and remain active in their community. The process of making the song is described in Chapter 6.

It is also important to recognise that finding voice is not only about standing up and speaking. The most important step is the first step taken and this is often the gesture of inviting someone to listen. The first step into a hospice. The first session with an art worker. Overcoming frailty and fear is complex and in Chapter 5 I outline ways of using non-verbal communication – movement and dance – to overcome fear and to accept support. This process relies on a transformation in the audience and the listener. We have to learn to listen to frailty and to reach out and support the performer. We have to learn to connect. We need to be open to different forms of art to enable people to perform themselves safely. Support is essential and the second part of the book is dedicated to Developing support.

Working with support groups is a well-established way to build structures for user involvement. Developing users groups and users forums has been very successful in mental healthcare where mental health service users have become active stakeholders in their places of care. In several mental health day centres service users not only sit actively on trustee boards but are also involved in the operational management of the centre. At Chelsea and Westminster Hospital, mental health service users have been active in recruitment and often sit on recruitment boards for new members of staff, including consultants and psychiatrists.

However, in chronic illness, terminal illness and life threatening conditions the role of service users is more complex. While a mental health diagnosis is often a lifelong condition, it is not always life threatening. People have a lifelong investment in the delivery of the service. A life threatening diagnosis is distinct. People either face a terminal diagnosis at the end of their life where frailty, and debility make active and useful functioning on trustee boards not necessarily effective, or people experience a life threatening diagnosis and recover after surgical intervention (HIV/AIDS, breast cancer, prostate cancer, for example). In these instances the most effective support can be collective through the formation of user groups that enable people to express feelings with safety. As is effectively pointed out in Chapter 9, support groups are not so much about activism for change as enabling people to find a safe space to be themselves without being judged. Support groups offer the safety of a confidential space without judgement. Some people may find voice within a support group and then want to make a public statement to deliver change. The work of Francesca Beard with a group of women who attended St Johns Hospice outlined in the second part of Chapter 10 pays tribute to this process and the group of women she worked with performed their work live on stage at Riverside Studios in 2004 and then they went on to collaborate with Francesca Beard in the writing of a play for broadcast on BBC Radio. A collective voice is an effective vehicle for strategic change. It enables a representative group to make clear public statements. However, it is important to realise that while a collective voice is useful for effective delivery of change, users forums, users groups are not always appropriate sites for activism. Support is not always synonymous with confidence and is not necessarily part of the development of a clear sense of personal or political identity.

The strategic bridge between finding identity, developing support and advancing involvement is not straightforward. In Chapter 7 Nuala Cullen and David Alcock explore some of the complex ideas that finding voice and identity pose to an individual hospice and look at the challenges St Andrew's Hospice faced when adopting the ideas and principles of good creative practice and of user involvement. At its most simple the role of personal storytelling has a direct impact on the new developments of narrative based medicine. Narrative is important in medicine because it performs a 'bridging' function that enables doctors (and other healthcare professionals) to travel across this bridge, taking the patient's story of illness and repackaging it in the form of a case history. It is important to involve the patient in this process and allow the story to travel to and fro in conversation so that the patient's story is kept alive. In principle, this means that a healthcare professional needs to allow the patient the time to tell their story. Sometimes people become trapped within their story of illness. Attentive listening enables a doctor to offer a different story to enable a patient, who sees themselves as passive victim, to become transformed, to see themselves as active participant in their narrative, changing the words that the doctor has given and finding their own language and their own story. The development of narrative based medicine is a good example of how doctors and patients can collaborate in the development of simple strategies to build bridges between finding voice and user involvement. If the doctor can give the patient enough time to tell the story and find their voice, the patient becomes an active participant in the delivery of their care. In this way, both doctor and patient educate each other and teach each other how to communicate.

In Chapter 12 doctors Emma Hall and Jennifer Todd outline ways in which patients have been involved in the training of medical students. This offers a clear way forward for the development of the art of storytelling within conventional medicine. These users groups are dependent upon the confident voice of the service user and sufficient support networks.

In Chapter 13 Sue Eckstein outlines a drama project that began with a group at St Christopher's and explores some of the ethical issues that surround how the group contributed to the final public piece of writing. This group is one where growing support and compatibility are the outcome of a creative group and where a confident support group contributed to the public voice. This development of public art shifts the practice from within the fabric of healthcare to public art. In this realm the art has a clear activist agenda.

The ethics of ownership and copyright become complex when an artist takes respon-sibility for the development of a work out of a collective process. These ethics still need debating in public and within traditional healthcare if the confident voice of the service user is to remain at the forefront of the agenda. Politically, it gives people the courage to voice themselves and it is important that the voice of the artist is one of collaborator and not interpreter if this political activism is to develop a significant voice in our culture.

One of the most significant developments is the potential of the internet to offer a creative and unmediated voice for service users. Julian Stallabrass has outlined the democ-ratic principles of internet art and these principles remain intact despite international censorship laws. The MS Society website offers message board forums where service users can explore issues from new diagnosis to everyday living, and message board forums targeted to young people, carers as well as people living with MS. In Chapter 14 we look at current online strategies to enable people to communicate their voices and ideas and the implications of the internet and new technologies for developing user support and involvement strategies. The last part of the book looks at models of good practice. Poems for World Day was an online initiative that invited service users and staff from across the world to submit poetry for an anthology published on World Day. The initiative was designed to find the voices of the national and international community and support this voice through the forum provided by the website. Chapter 16 is a bold look at how to use service user forums to challenge the culture of gratiude within the hoospice movement and the last chapter of the book pays tribute to the views, stories and direct experiences of the members of the Help the Hospices service user involvement initiative.

First and foremost, the book is intended to be a good read. A survey of how people are tackling these ideas and some of the measures being introduced. It is dedicated to Paul Laking, a very good friend. In 1999 I stayed in his family home in Suffolk while running a residency at St Nicholas Hospice, Bury St Edmunds and was welcomed into his home and family. He became involved in the stories that I was listening to and came to the celebration event that marked the end of the residency. A couple of years later he became involved in a short video drama we produced in collaboration with bereaved teenagers, where he played the father to the lead character. Three years later he was diagnosed with secondary cancer in his liver and died several weeks later. I lent him a video camera he used to record stories for his family and also suggested he wrote some poems and explored his own lyricism. He emailed them to me and they preface each section of the book. His final text was sent to my phone a week before he died. He was watching fireworks over the Suffolk coast and was amazed at the brilliance of the fireworks and the intensity of his experience of life as he faced death. He loved life and had an incredible curiosity that enabled him to get involved in almost everything that intrigued him. His poems invite you to listen and understand his perspective of living with a terminal illness. I hope you will be inspired by this and the other stories you read and be encouraged to get involved yourself.

Lucinda Jarrett
August 2007

About the editor

Lucinda Jarrett is artistic director of Rosetta Life, an artist-led organisation that delivers artist-led residencies in hospices and hospitals across England. She founded the organisation in 1997 in order to challenge our contemporary representation of illness and to enable people who are facing death to participate more fully in cultural life.

Lucinda read English Literature and Theatre at Edinburgh University and then studied the semiotics of dance at the University of Paris. She worked in television for five years where she worked as assistant television producer for French, American and British broadcasters, and has written and performed performance poetry across London venues. She is a published writer and has worked with independent dance venues and independent dancers and has a strong track record of delivering theatre within healthcare settings.

List of contributors

Suzy Croft is a senior social worker at St John's Palliative Care Centre and Research Fellow at the Centre for Citizen Participation at Brunel University.

Peter Beresford OBE is Professor of Social Policy and Director of the Centre for Citizen Participation at Brunel University. He is also Chair of Shaping Our Lives: the national user network. He is a long-term user of mental health services and active in the mental health service users/survivors movement.

Chapter 1
Chris Rawlence is a film maker, writer and librettist. Since 2001 he has been working with Rosetta Life where he is an artist in residence at Greenwich and Bexley Cottage Hospice.

Chapter 2
Heidi Morstang is an artist specialising in photography and the moving image.

Dr Elizabeth Shafford has worked in child health and paediatrics with 20 years' experience in the field of paediatric oncology. She now works part time at St Luke's Hospice, Basildon.

Margarita was a service user of St Luke's Hospice, Basildon.

Chapter 3
Katherine Vaughan-Williams was an influential architectural historian and writer. She adored 1960s radio comedy and PG Wodehouse who inspired this work. Katherine died in September 2003.

Chapter 4
Marielle Macleman studied drawing and painting at Duncan of Jordanstone College of Art and Design, Dundee and now co-ordinates the arts project at the Prince and Princess of Wales Hospice, Glasgow.

John Lieser was diagnosed with cancer in 1999 and given a prognosis of weeks. He was referred to the Prince and Princess of Wales Hospice, Glasgow where he is an active service user.

Chapter 5
Lucinda Jarrett is an artist who works with words, moving images and performance.

Miranda Tufnell has been working as a dancer and choreographer since 1976. She has also trained in Alexander Technique and craniosacral therapy.

Chapter 6
Billy Bragg, is an English musician renowned for his blend of folk, punk-rock and protest music. He has been active for over 20 years.

Maxine Edgington was a service user at Trimar Hospice, Weymouth. She died in March 2006.

Catherine Batten is Rosetta Life artist in residence at Trimar Hospice, Weymouth. She also works with West Dorset Food and Land Trust where she co-ordinates the Bridport Local Food Heritage Project.

Chapter 7
Nuala Cullen is the Principal Family Support Worker at St Andrew's Hospice, Grimsby.

David Alcock is the Creative Therapy Co-ordinator at St Andrew's Hospice, Grimsby.

Chapter 8
Gillian Chowns is a Senior Lecturer in Palliative Care at Oxford Brookes University and a former Specialist Palliative Care Social Worker with the East Berks Macmillan Palliative Care Team.

Sue Bussey is a Specialist Palliative Care Social Worker with the East Berks Macmillan Palliative Care Team.

Alison Jones is a former Principal Social Worker with Thames Hospice Care and was instrumental in setting up their Bereavement Service. She is a qualified counsellor and since her retirement has worked as a supervisor and trainer for Cruse Bereavement Care.

Nick Lunch has been an enthusiastic advocate and pioneer of participatory video (PV) techniques for 10 years and is Director of Insight (www.insightshare.org).

Chapter 9
The women who use the St Thomas's Hospital support group are living with breast cancer or need support as a result of breast cancer treatment.

Chapter 10
Suzy Croft and the St John's Hospice Women's Support Group and Francesca Beard.

Chapter 11
Phil Cotterall is a Research Fellow in Palliative Care at Worthing and Southlands Hospitals NHS Trust.

Chapter 12

Dr Emma Hall is Consultant in Palliative Medicine, St Christopher's Hospice, London.

Dr Jennifer Todd is Consultant in Palliative Medicine, Trinity Hospice, London.

Chapter 13

Sue Eckstein works at the Centre of Medical Law and Ethics, King's College London, where she is currently Director of Programme Development, specialising in ethical issues in medical research.

Bobbie Farsides has been teaching and researching in the field of bioethics for almost 20 years. In July 2006 she moved to a new post at the Brighton and Sussex Medical School where she holds the Foundation Chair in Clinical and Biomedical Ethics.

Chapter 14 and 15

Lucinda Jarett is an artist who works with words, moving images and performances.

Chapter 16

Judith Hodgson is the Senior Lecturer in Psychosocial and Education Services at Dove House Hospice, the Vice Chair of the Association of Palliative Care Social Workers and a Trustee of Help the Hospices.

Chapter 17

Suzy Croft, Peter Beresford, Munir Lanani, Di Cowdrey, Mandy Paine, Karen Willman, David Hart and **Anne Macfarlane**: Help the Hospices' User Involvement Initiative.

PART 1: FINDING A VOICE

My Place at the Front of the Queue

I know my place
I'm the one without the luggage
The big adventure at the front of my view.
Sure of my place in the queue.
Looking back at people
Things we've done
Excited by the prospects
New experiences or none
Part of the biosphere or a golden plover on Ixworth water meadow?
Can't look at that now.
Got to look to make sure they they know
Where the spare wheel is
How to make bread
How to change records on the jukebox
Who to call when the computer plays silly buggers
All not-mes doing my job
Love-you-and-leave-you
Hugs a little longer
Kisses nearer to on the lips
Looks full of meaning
'How could you go, you bastard?'
'How could you? How could you?'
When you gotta go, you gotta go, babe
Journey to the Indies
Sail off into the sunset
On red tsunamis.
Beauty and Death.
Love and rockets.

Paul Laking
1 January 2005

CHAPTER 1

John's song

Chris Rawlence

I am a filmmaker, photographer and writer. I collaborate with people facing terminal illness and together we make films, write songs and poems, or take photographs about things that matter. The process is about the creative empowerment of those whom life-threatening illness has disempowered. It is about the resurrection of voices that have been silenced by illness. The outcome of these collaborations is, for want of a less pretentious word, art – and, if the person wishes, this is often presented at public events and shared on the internet.

Over the past five years I have been midwife to over fifty short films, and numerous songs, poems, and photoworks made in this way. Many of these projects have taken place at Greenwich and Bexley Cottage Hospice in South-East London. Here is the story of one of them – a song – and the man whose love story it describes.

1 September 2004

Hi Chris, It's me again, I am sorry to bother you. But I am going grey haired trying to figure out how to get on rosettalife email, I just don't know what more I can do. What am I doing wrong? I want to put these photos on my file at the hospice. Do you have any ideas? I know you must be busy. So just when you have time. Be lucky. Big John.

John, Check your e-mails from me – I told you that you won't get on to your own rosetta life e-mail because we're still sorting it. Instead, use your own – the one you e-mailed me with. As for the rosettalife website that I suggested you go into – well, it's the same as ever – so check out www.rosettalife.org then go to Community for the Paul poems I suggested you look at. As for gray hair, well at least you have some growing again that is able to go gray. Only joking! Computers can drive a person – including me – MAD, can't they. But they keep us alert!!! Chris.

3 November 2004

A large man with a feathery looking crew cut is watching me move stuff around in iPhoto on one of the Macs we have down here at the hospice. I watch him from the corner of my eye, waiting for the opportunity to turn and engage him in the conversation that I know he's itching to have with me. He's one of a group of elderly men sitting round a table in the day centre of the hospice. The others are eyeing the drinks trolley, which is clinking over from the other side of the room, but John wants to ask me about computers.

He is breathless today, inhaling short sips of air as he makes his way towards me. And I'm cross, he tells me in a broad Scottish accent, because I've been up half the night trying to organise my photos on the computer I've just bought myself, but something went wrong and I don't know whether I've lost the photos, or accidentally put them somewhere I can't find them. Basically he doesn't know where the hell they are and he's pissed off. So I make a few suggestions as to where he might find them, reassure him that he's not the only one to be driven mad by a computer and then, annoyingly no doubt, I suggest that the best learning happens through making mistakes and no, he's not stupid, we all make mistakes, particularly with new software. Maybe I should pay you a visit, I suggest, and we could solve the problem together.

15 November 2004

John lives in a small council flat in South-East London. His living room is skimpily furnished. He greets me from his armchair, surrounded by the paraphernalia of lung cancer – oxygen machine, mask, pills. Next to him, on a sofa, his tiny silver-haired wife Gina sits quietly with a bemused smile watching a muted episode of Bargain Hunt on a large telly. And the computer.

'I found the photos Chris', he says sheepishly. 'They were sitting there on the desktop all the time. I'm sorry to have dragged you out here now. What a fool!'

'No worries,' I say. 'It's what I do,' because actually I have come for reasons other than John's lost photographs although he doesn't yet know this.

Perhaps I shouldn't have been surprised when one of the volunteers at the hospice told me that John had had a professional career as a singer and an actor. I discovered that he'd been a truck driver when, one evening, after a particularly bad performance by a singer at a working men's club he shouted out, 'I could do better than that!' The MC rounded on him at once, 'There's a fella here thinks he can sing!' And he could. He gave up his day job and for the next twenty years made a reasonable living from the club circuit and Old Time Music Hall, and then parts in musicals on the London stage.

This unlikely singing career peaked at the Lyceum in the Strand, where he was topping the bill when a BBC Producer offered him a part in *Porridge*. 'I couldn'a stand the idea of singing love songs beyond my sell by,' John said. 'So I took the job.' Lots of television followed - mostly character parts in shows like *Hitchhiker's Guide*, and *Yellowbeard, Our Friends in the North*. Then came the feature films – parts in *Batman* and *Hear My Song*.

John's lung cancer was diagnosed in 2003, when he was 70. As is so often the case, serious illness struck on retirement. His hopes for a life of relaxation and ease were cruelly shot down by a terminal diagnosis. I met him a year later, by which time his shock and distress had receded – and so too had the modest celebrity of his career. John seemed to be back where he had started – a small council flat and no obvious wealth.

It's the fact that John has been a singer that appeals to me. Rosetta Life are currently producing an ambitious online project called the Rosetta Requiem. It's a cycle of 12 songs and 6 short films, that is being made in collaborations between people like John, who have a terminal illness, and known composers, filmmakers, songwriters. The idea is to turn the traditional idea of the Requiem on its head – to celebrate the lives of those that are still here rather than grieve for those who have gone. Now if I could get John to work with me on the lyrics of a song, match him with a songwriter, and maybe even get him to sing it – that would be something – and it's this that I'll broach with him today as we troubleshoot his computer.

Part of my job involves watching out for the salient in what people are saying. I listen and probe gently, then listen some more. Often I have my laptop open and type in the stream of words as they emerge. Sometimes I can't keep up and only the significant gets jotted down. It's like panning for gold must have been. Together we sieve through the rubble, on the lookout for the glint in what remains. Today, it's an event rather than John's words that catches my attention. Or rather, a non-event, because as we've been chatting

I've become aware that John's wife, Gina, has been oddly passive. She has been watching me with a strange politeness and as we finish John asks her to make us a cup of tea. She seems pleased to have something to do and vanishes into the kitchen with an air of purpose. Later I compliment her on the tea and notice something about her expression. It is as if she has not fully understood me and is scared of asking me what I mean. She seems to have forgotten why I'm here or who I am.

20 November 2004
At the hospice today John explains. 'Dementia' is the word he uses.
   'Alzheimer's?' I ask, and he nods.

25 February 2005
It's been a while since my visit to John and the difficulty of his situation has stayed with me. Nothing has yet happened with the song I envisaged, but we've been in regular contact because he is very keen to have his own page on the Rosetta Life web site, where he can post his own photographs and thoughts, and share his experience with others. The idea of these community pages is that hospice users can add content to their own small part of the web site, thereby gaining a degree of control over the process, but there's still a modest digital learning curve involved and this – like the e-mails – has frustrated John, who needs results – now.

What strikes me about John's enthusiasm for digital technology is that it allows him to bring some order to a life that feels to him as if it's disintegrating. Simple photo applications, message boards, and word processing, enable him to discover sense in his own story and tell it to others. A terminal diagnosis – no euphemisms here because that's what it is – is a seriously destabilising event in a person's life. This much is obvious but what's not so apparent is the traumatic disempowerment and decentering that comes with it. Where once your identity turned on your job status and position at the centre of the family, now you are best known for your illness – a depressed drag, without voice, on those around you. All the old certainties fragment as the world you knew flies apart.

The situation is, literally, chronic. In many cases it won't be curtailed by sudden death. These days a terminal diagnosis is likely to mean several years living with incurable illness. But although you may be disabled, in pain, and coping with the side effects of medication, you may still be able to live a moderately active life and will probably want to do so. Terminal illness is as much about living life differently as it is about the business of death and dying. An unsolicited encounter with mortality faces us all with the big questions and fears, but it also offers us the chance to re-evaluate priorities. And this often involves 'getting things in order'.

Humans seem to like things in order, whether as babies putting shapes into boxes or as partially sighted adults with a brain tumour cementing mosaic tiles to the frame of a mirror that will be sold in the hospice handicraft shop. Particularly we like to combat the disorder of illness by ordering, be it through painting by numbers, a computer photo-application, an online chat room, or a song. The mosaic mirror provides a tiny purchase on a world that is slipping away, the controlled manipulation of a thing that gratifies the instinct to transform. Photo-applications, song-writing, or blogging are among those creative activities that raise the ordering instinct to a higher level, from simple arrangement to the organisation of a life's events into something that offers cohesion and meaning – a story.

Today we're talking about computers again and I decide to ask John about his home situation. We retreat to the privacy of a side room and I pull out the laptop. I ask him how things are at home. The words come pouring out, slowed only by his gasps for breath. He speaks about the love and frustration of his life with Gina. On the face of things they complement each other: John in total command of his mental faculties but physically disabled by the dreadful breathlessness of lung cancer; Gina – 'fit as a fiddlers flea' but some way along the mind-devastating journey that is Alzheimer's Disease. There's an awful neatness to their contrasting incapacities. 'I am her brain', John says. 'But while I sit in the bath she pours water over me, she brews a cup of tea, she does the physical things I am no longer able to.'

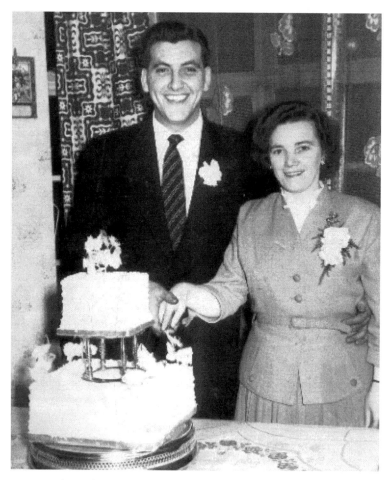

FIGURE 1 John and Gina on their wedding day.

I become more alert. I've glimpsed the flash of gold I'm on the lookout for, the salient experience, the core of what might become an extraordinary song. As John talks I press him for detail while typing continuously. This is the heart of the collaborative creative process. All my faculties are now focused on sifting the stream of John's words for what matters. I ask nosey questions, I prompt, I tease, and listen, as he speaks. He trusts me. When we're done I've filled four pages with what seems to matter and this pivots on the role of the carer and cared-for. We arrange to talk more. Meanwhile, I will try to shape his words into the lyrics of a song.

What's going on here? What right have I to decide what is salient? Whose voice is emerging? Are we both the lyricist? Am I the facilitator? A therapist? This is tricky terrain but worth crossing for the light that it sheds on the meaning of the phrase 'user led' and the nature of collaborative process. To begin with, I have pride, a craftsman's pride in my skill for writing librettos and, from time to time, the lyrics of a song. My skill here lies first in listening, then in selecting and raising the lyrical vernacular that is John's way of speaking into the form of a poem or song that is true to his experience. It entails the shunting and rearrangement of phrases and the discovery of John's authentic voice in the new shape that is emerging. It requires complete truth to the exchanges that occurred between us, no embellishment. It involves recognising what is dross and discarding it.

For example, in the flow of speaking about Gina's Alzheimer's John had said:

> 'When friends ask how I am, she'll say I'm up the pub with friends, like in the old days, when I am just out in the garden. I couldna' draw breath but I was down the pub. What makes it bearable is that you've got to laugh. She'll ask, What's the day – a 100 times a day. I'm getting more and more impatient and when I get upset it upsets her. Rather than say some thing, I just say OK. Yesterday I had a bath, but I canna get in or out of a bath. Gina runs the bath for me. I sit on the bath edge and Gina pours the water over me. She still does that. She'll rub my back and dry my feet. She gets pleasure from this. It makes her feel wanted. She pulls my socks on for me. She's always says, I did this for my father. She's my body but I have to be her brain. I've made arrangements for the future. She's well looked after if anything happens to me. My daughter is her carer too. My concern is that when I go will she get any worse? But once I kick the bucket there's nothing I can do. The best scenario would be if she would pass on first. But she's fit as a fiddler's flea.'

Sitting at home, I take great care to preserve John's actual words and turns of phrase. Whatever emerges from this process has to feel authentic and true to him. Catching the texture and rhythm of his speech is crucial. Because of the rich simplicity of John's imagery and the colloquiality of his speech, the shaping comes easily. First, the fulcrum of the lyric emerges – 'You be my body, darling. Let me be your brain.' Then everything else seems to fall into place, radiating from that kernel of a chorus line. It's not always this simple. The end result is long, too long for a song, but a great starting point.

20 March 2005

Dear John, I've had a go at what we worked on – here it is. I've tried to enfold what you said into the structure of a song – that you might sing?? Nothing's final with this. I've taken a few liberties. Let me know what feels right or wrong, what else you'd like to see. It's up to you to tell me what is true. When we get the words right, then we'll find a musician, or three. This is a draft. I think we can find a more affirmative ending. Hope you've had a good Easter and I'll be in contact mid week. Chris

> My wife is fit, fit as a fiddler's flea
> I'll sit on the bath as she pours water over me

What day is it today?
You've got to laugh
What day is it today?
Again and again, the same refrain
You be my body, darling
Let me be your brain

You are still beautiful
I'm still your loving John
But some things that we had are gone

She's fit, still brews a cup of tea
I canna draw breath but she'll pull on my socks for me
What day is it today?
The Dance of Death
What day is it today?
We'll sing the same refrain
You be my body, darling
Let me be your brain

25 March 2005
Hi Chris, Well, what can I say, I honestly think what you have done is brilliant, I have trouble reading it for the tears blurring my vision, I find it very moving. As you have captured my feelings so exact. Keep happy, Big John.

I'm thrilled, of course, that John likes the song but something is niggling me. I was so excited by the neatness of the line 'You be my body darling, Let me be your brain' that I knowingly put other words into John's mouth and when we next meet he raises this. He reiterates his delight in the song but there's one line he'd like changed. In the second verse, as an internal rhyme to 'I canna draw breath', I have written 'The Dance of Death'. Even as I wrote this I knew that I was taking a liberty because John had not actually said it. Now, as we speak about it, he feels that line is too maudlin – this is a love song, not a death song. So there and then we change the line to 'What time is left?' – keeping the rhyme while still alluding to mortality but without the directness of what often gets called 'the D word' in hospices.

27 March 2005
Marion, Artist-in-Residence at St Christopher's Hospice, has paid a visit to Greenwich and Bexley Hospice where I introduce her to John. He shows her his pages on the Community Site – a brief life story, some photographs and poems. Marion tells John about Paul, a Jamaican man, she is working with. Paul, who has cancer and is blind, has been moved from the hospice to a nursing home where he's now feeling very isolated and wants to make contact with someone – anyone – about his situation. Marion shows us the pages she has set up for Paul on the Community Site and invites John to make contact.

Paul's web page is a vehicle for his poetry. It's also his window on the world, even though he's blind. This troubled and talented man reaches sightlessly out to us from his pillow in the thumbnail photograph on the page. In the right bar are the titles of his poems, one of which we open with a click.

There's a game I play inside my head
Pretending that I am already dead
Just to be here to see
Those I've left behind me
Friends and lovers weeping
While I lie here sleeping
Some will never recall
I was ever here at all
And others will laugh out of hand
Or say I was a good kind man
While thinking deep inside
I was base, low and snide.
Who in this darkness
Who will hear my plea?
Who will remember me as me?

In the left bar of Paul's page there's a long vertical branch with coloured fruit-like dots hanging from it. A click on each fruit brings up a message from someone who's read Paul's poems and wants to communicate with him. John is very keen to say something. The whole notion of using the internet to connect with others going through similar experiences excites him, so we add a message.

Dear Paul, I have just read your poems, and was greatly moved by them, you have a great talent and a gift to make words come to life. More, more, more. Please may I thank you most sincerely. Be Lucky. Big John Dair

A few days later we add another—

Hi Paul, Its John Dair again just to say how much I enjoyed the new poems on your page, what a talent you have Paul, and now a favour to ask, I have dabbled with words on my page and would be delighted if you would have a look and maybe advice me on how I am doing, but don't be too cruel, ha ha. My best wishes Paul, please keep up the good work, A Big Fan. John Dair

Breath in, breath out, breath in, breath out.
Three score years and ten,
I can't remember when I had
Trouble breathing in and breathing out.
I mean it is so easy, the natural thing to do.
That is until some illness befalls you.

By now John has copied me into these exchanges.

John, I like your Breathing text. Let's go to work on it and discover its rhythm, its pulse, its breath ... and make a song of this as well. I aim to be in next Monday so hope to see you then. Chris

John and Paul's correspondence continues for a few weeks, helped at each end by Marion and myself. John seems to thrive on the communication, pleased to be helping someone else. At first they stick to e-mail but then Marion arranges for Paul to record one of his poems with a message that can be uploaded to our server, and then downloaded by John to his computer at home. John is pleased when this works – proud that he actually managed to download it and warmed by the closeness to Paul that hearing his voice engenders. But it's a short-lived relationship because Marion calls the next day to say that Paul has died.

1 April 2005

People often ask me how I cope with the steady loss of those with whom I work. I don't know how you do it, they might say. So many relationships gone, just like that. And I answer that maybe it takes a certain kind of person to work with the dying, that we workers in palliative care share a benign battlezone aptitude that allows us to give hugely without ever letting those to whom we are giving come too close. A subtly defended generosity of spirit that allows us to move out and move on as the daily reality of a hospice demands. True, the constant presence of death can sap energy and depress. Dying, by definition, is a process of waning energy and sometimes I wake up with distinct feeling that I do not want to go to that fusty death place today, the place of wheelchairs, incontinence, fear, pain, desperation. But then I drive to the hospice and these forebodings disperse and I get down to the creative business of panning for gold with those who are dying and have become, yes, my friends. We dig down into life to discover meaning. We write poems and song lyrics, we make movies and take photographs together and find that the release of creative energy works against the downward direction of dying. For a limited period of time – a few weeks, months, sometimes a year or two – the dying person will rediscover themselves, find their voice, and make a beautiful thing.

This unexpected late flowering of personality and skill, and the repossession of self that comes with it, can have remarkable consequences. On several occasions I've noticed that creative collaboration has an analgesic effect. People who are dependent on high doses of morphine to alleviate pain may find that they don't need the drug for the few hours a week that they are absorbed creatively. Rather than simple distraction – or diversion – this seems to be the positive outcome of creative engagement. Artists sometimes refer to the act of making as 'getting your juices flowing' and maybe they are sensing a neurochemical emotional reality here that can actually raise the pain threshold for those living with cancer.

The effect of a creative collaboration that lasts several months is cumulative. A person – John, say – will discover the creative instinct that may have been flattened by illness or lain dormant within him for many years. The delight in this discovery leads to the making of amazing things and the energising of personality. In the flow towards death we are perhaps building little islands of artistic assertion that work against the current. For a while, hopefully, a person re-enters life with a transformed sense of self, having re-evaluated what matters. And this will be communicated to family, friends, and the hospice community, through artwork, but also through personality.

Not that we make miracle claims for art, or raise what we do above the spectrum of counselling, alternative therapies, spiritual guidance, and good medical care that makes most hospices exceptional places. Nor are we in denial about the nature of death and its cold finality – who wants it!

1 June 2005

John's Song is one of these islands in the current and we're still building it. I have decided to introduce him to the composer Orlando Gough, with a view to Orlando setting the lyrics we have written. I take Orlando to John's flat and we sit out in the garden surrounded by pots of Busy Lizzies that John delights in photographing and uploading to his webpage. Orlando particularly likes the lines You be my body darling, Let me be your brain. It's a gift for a composer, he says. In fact I love the whole song, even if it is a bit long.

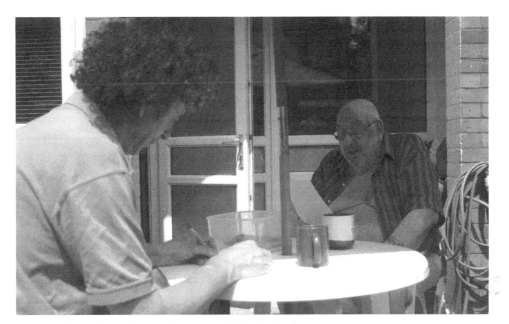

FIGURE 2 John Dair working with composer Orlando Gough.

We chat on. John is keen to tell Orlando how impressed he is with a healer at the hospice who by laying on hands has immediately released the sick weight he's been feeling across his chest. And not only this – he has somehow managed to relax his wife Gina – at a distance. They'd been arguing a lot and Gina's Alzheimer's was leading her to make all sorts of annoying accusations – like John eating the last donut. Most frustrating of all were her mantras – What day is it today? What time is it? – lines that had now found their way into the song – Day after day, the same refrain, you be my body darling, let me be your brain.

This has its funny side. You've got to laugh, John says, but it's also been driving me crazy. Yet somehow this healer has helped her by working on me. I was an old cynic, but I can't deny what this guy has achieved.

It's obvious from our visit that John will not have the energy or breath to sing his own song, which is sad but he's the first to acknowledge it. This seems to be part of the general movement towards acceptance that I have observed in him. In fact he told me last week that the doctors have advised against any further chemo and operating on his lung is now out of the question. His concern now is not so much for himself as for Gina, whose Alzheimer's can only get worse. He needs to feel that she will be properly looked after when he's gone.

Time to leave. Orlando will set the song for Martin, a singer he frequently works with through his choir, The Shout. We will present the song at a celebration event at the hospice in ten days time, so there's no time to lose, particularly if John is to hear the song before the day.

7 July 2005
It's gone to the fence. It's now noon on the day of the event that is due to start at 2.00. John has arrived early. Not only has he not yet heard the song but Martin hasn't rehearsed

it. It's just as well that John is a singer and – being an old pro – knows from experience how much is brought together at the last minute. He watches from the other side of the room as Jonathan accompanies Martin's first efforts on the piano. After a few false starts Martin gets in to the flow and John likes what he hears. They stop to discuss a line and John suggests a small change that Orlando is happy to incorporate.

Celebration Events are highpoints of a Rosetta Life residency. Typically, the Rosetta Life artist – who at Greenwich and Bexley Cottage Hospice is myself – may have worked with up to 30 people in the preceding months – both as individuals and in groups – to make a video, write a poem or a story, or take photographs about something that matters to them. The Event, which will have been well publicised and prepared for, is an opportunity for people to present their work to their friends and families, and to the wider hospice community. They are often emotional affairs, in which people rather than their conditions shine through. Today is no exception. There are 40 people here, including the deputy mayor.

There are several songs on the programme – the fruit of other Rosetta Life collaborations between musicians and people like John. There are also some videos and two poems, performed by their authors.

When we reach John's Song, John himself introduces it.

'Hello,' he begins. 'My name is John Dair and I'm an alcoholic. Whoops! Wrong meeting.' There's laughter at this and this gets John into his stride as a performer. For a moment we might be back in the working men's club where his singing career began. 'I'd never have thought that I'd find myself back in the music business,' he jokes. 'But I am, and here's the result. It's a love song.'

Martin starts singing, entrancing the audience with the gentle pathos of the song. I can't quite tell whether the gradual heaving of John's chest is due to his breathlessness or because he's crying, but when he pulls out a tissue and dabs at an eye I realise that the event is almost – but not quite – too much for him.

There are differing schools of thought about prompting powerful emotion at hospice social events. Rosetta have hosted some presentations at which families have wept openly in response to seeing their loved ones on video or watching them perform. Sometimes hospice support staff feel that such outpourings are unduly upsetting, not just for those weeping but also for other bereaved families who might be in the audience. Surely, they've argued, the support group or one-to-one counselling session is the place for expressing these feelings – not a public social event where there's no obvious safety net and people will go home full of painful unresolved emotion.

Watching John weep reminds me of these arguments. I realise that I could be deemed irresponsible for making his poignant personal situation – Gina's Alzheimer's and his cancer – so public. Yet I know that we're doing the right thing here and we should not be afraid. How do I know? Intuition is the simple answer, a gut instinct that possibly serves my judgement better than a counselling qualification or a therapy diploma. Not that I take issue with the need for professional alertness in this kind of situation, or the need for training; it's more that I am wary of those professional protocols that may close down rather than open up events, leading to an over protective approach in which too little is risked. I suppose this comes down to personality and judgement but I have never yet been involved in a Rosetta event which families regretted attending or participating in, however much they wept. There is lasting applause when the song is over. John, dry eyed now, turns to acknowledge the audience with a broad grin.

13 September 2005
We are recording John's Song at Angel Studios in Islington. My friend Keith, from the hospice, has driven John all the way from Plumstead to be here. Keith also has lung cancer, but that's another story.

Orlando has arranged the song for accordion, bass, bass clarinet and piano – an instrumentation that brings out John's Scottishness, particularly the pipey cry of the accordion. The music is evocative and I find myself picturing John and Gina being rowed the length of a Scottish loch, their figures silhouetted against the blue water and the mountains beyond – all very romantic but almost certainly too cheesy for the video that I will make to accompany the song on the website.

Halfway through the recording John signals that wants to leave. I've noticed his breathlessness and can see that he's anxious. My plan was to rush him down the road to University College Hospital if there had been a problem but John must go now. He's right. The anxiety brought on by breathlessness creates more breathlessness, and more anxiety – a vicious circle – and there's no nebuliser in this studio.

20 October 2005
John hasn't been at the hospice for four weeks and I'm concerned about his health. When I call I hear the breathlessness in his voice. He's been in hospital with a chest infection and is now home for a while. He's not sure that he'll have the energy to come to the hospice next week so I decide to pay him a visit.

I have a feeling that John is on his home run. After this unexpected creative burst through the summer months, he is now declining, like the seasonal arc of the year. I don't think he'll make it through to Christmas and I alert the hospice to his situation.

31 October 2005
I bumped into John being wheeled into the hospice this morning. He was hooked up to an oxygen cylinder and drowsy from morphine. I placed my palm over the back of his hand and we acknowledged wordlessly that he is nearing the end. Later I visited him in his room and woke him gently from his druggy sleep. He was not in pain but very low on energy. I got the DVD Chris – it's just wonderful, he whispered, with what seemed enormous effort.

5 November 2005
John has been moved to another room, on the sunny side of the hospice, and it's much better than the dark room he has left, which felt a bit like a mausoleum. I find him sitting, slightly slumped, in a chair next to his bed. He acknowledges me with a slight upward movement of his head.

I sit down opposite him and lean in closely, the better to catch something he's trying to say. With my ear a few centimetres from his mouth I hear him say softly 'I've made arrangements for Gina. I just hope that she'll be OK.'

6 April 2006
The path I accompanied John on, though unique, shares a pattern with many of the journeys I've made with people who are dying. The person I first encounter may be angry and depressed, but as the weeks go by their involvement with Rosetta affects their countenance. Pessimism gives way to more openness, excitement even, as they discover aspects of themselves that they had long forgotten about. The freeing up of cramped creativity, the waking of the making instinct that in most of us has lain dormant since childhood, is

pivotal to this transformation. The recognition and embrace of self that creativity ushers in is a healing event – not in its unlikely ability to shrink tumours or reverse neuro-degenerative disease but in the new lease of life, sometimes stretching to years, that may come about.

And yet ... and yet ... is this anything more than a temporary reprieve? Like our English year with its summer that ends, if we're lucky, with one of those glorious Indian summers in September – a grand finale that is all too soon shoved aside by October gales that rip the dry leaves from the trees in the darkening afternoons. It's then that you wonder whether summer had ever happened, just as the death of someone with whom you have worked closely may lead you to ask yourself whether the whole trip was worth it.

But such feelings are sent packing when you receive e-mails like this, picked up at an internet café when, recently, I was defying the English winter on holiday in Barbados.

Hello, I'm writing to see if it would be possible to put the song your wonderful charity did with my Dad on to a DVD. Sadly he passed away last November and I was unaware that he had been involved in the making of this song. I just happened to stumble on it when I was surfing the net.

It really was such a lovely thing to find and for him to have done with everyone's help. It's strange because I did read over Xmas about the lady who had written a song for her daughter with Billy Bragg but I had no idea that the same people had worked with my Dad.

I would be very grateful for anything you could send me. Steven Dair

This kind of message is a testament to the magic of the internet and its empowering potential. Unquestionably John benefited from his involvement with Rosetta Life in the course of his final year, and so did those around him. The quality of his life improved and with this he became a less testy, more giving, person. But the framing of his song on the internet, and the steadily increasing number of visits that the site is attracting, suggest that there is a dimension to this intimate personal work that also thrives in the public realm. What John and others in his position discover in themselves, and find the voice to express, matters to others. For me, exploring the dynamic relationship between the personal and the public arena is a central aspect of our work and renders occasional doubts I may have about whether it's all worth it insignificant.

8 April 2006

I have been thinking about John's wife Gina so I e-mailed Steven back. It was my realisation that she had Alzheimer's that sowed the initial seed of John's song. How was she now, I wondered.

Hi Chris, it's nice of you to ask about my Mum. Her health is good but her mind is getting worse by the week. She is forgetting our names and at times who we are. She is living with one of my sisters and my niece is caring for her during the day. They do an amazing job as at times she can be very difficult to deal with as well as the constant repeating herself. Nearly every day she asks us if we know that Dad has died, and then she says that her Dad has died as well. She makes that sound as if it were last week when in fact he died before I was born.

I know my sister will have my Mum as long as she knows where she is and who we are. When she stops we shall have to have a rethink about what to do. The main thing is that Mum is happy where she is for now –well, as much as she can remember.

Anyway, I just wanted to thank you again for all your time and for giving my Dad the opportunity to make his song. It's sad that it's often too late when it hits you just how talented people are. Steven Dair.

Chris Rawlence is a filmmaker, writer and librettist. For the past 20 years he has been a TV director of many documentaries, drama documentaries, and TV operas for BBC, C4 and foreign broadcasters. He is also a writer and librettist and published works include *The Missing Reel* (Collins 1990).

Since 2001 he has been working with Rosetta Life where he is an artist in residence at Greenwich and Bexley Cottage Hospice exploring what matters with the life-threatened through video, photography, writing and drama and is also video director – responsible for moving picture output of the company.

CHAPTER 2

Margarita's story

Heidi Morstang, Dr Elizabeth Shafford and Margarita

Margarita's creative journey during the three last months of her life

Heidi Morstang

When I was introduced to Margarita (80) she told me she wasn't able to cry although she felt she had a lot of tears inside. Every time someone had tried to work on this with her, she said she only got hiccups. Margarita's aim was to live until she was a hundred because she had so much to do. She wanted to write a book for every parent to read. Also she wanted to outlive her mother who had reached 96.

She told me this in day care at St Luke's Hospice in Basildon, where I worked as a Rosetta Life artist-in-residence. I was intrigued by her gentle and wise way of speaking, and her persona was captivating for everybody who entered the room. Somehow her presence gave calmness to the space, and I later realised the other hospice users approached her to share their problems.

During this initial conversation when I introduced Rosetta Life and offered her the chance to work in a creative way, she said she thought she wasn't able to, as she was losing her vision. Margarita appeared to have very little self-worth but when she told me what she had done in her life, I couldn't believe that she could have such low self-worth. Amongst the many things she had done was teaching pupils at a stage school. She still received letters from her former students, telling her how much she had done for them. She had also published books and had loved creative writing because it was a way of expressing her thoughts.

One of the first things she mentioned was that she wanted to tell her mother's story, but she didn't know why. She said her mother visited her as a ghost by sitting in the chair opposite her in her living room. Margarita felt she had to explore why she was still there. Her mother's presence seemed to be disturbing, as the ghost was looking at Margarita in a strict negative way, and Margarita felt angry at her because she wanted to 'get rid of her mother'. Margarita's sight was deteriorating and she missed reading and writing as much as she had done before. She had previously published books and poetry and would have liked to continue writing. However, she went home and drew the story of her mother with pencils.

She brought these drawings to the hospice the following week. They were colourful drawings depicting her mother's life as a child and teenager, when she was sent to a Carmelite convent and later to a big house as a servant. Margarita was not very pleased with the drawings, at least she said she wasn't. However, I was intrigued by them. I found the drawings expressive and realised Margarita must have spent a long time drawing them. This week, she also read a piece of prose she had written a few years ago. It had the title 'My Lovely Blue Lady', and she explained it was about her spiritual guide who had been with her throughout her life. When she read the piece, her voice was vibrant. She explained the lovely blue lady could not be described visually; the blue colour only existed as a spiritual colour.

That week, Rosetta Life had a celebration event in the hospice, where the hospice users could share their work with other hospice users, their families, friends, and staff. Margarita framed her drawings to put on display in the hospice and she also read 'My Lovely Blue Lady'. Although she appeared to struggle with reading due to her poor vision, she captivated the audience. It was a magical moment. Her words were powerful, and I think she transmitted the presence of the lovely blue lady to the audience. Weeks after the celebration event, other hospice users and staff mentioned the calmness it had created in them when Margarita had read it. When I mentioned this to her, she said she was worried that she could not pray for herself although she prayed for the other hospice users.

After the celebration event, several of the other hospice users made contact with Margarita and also started calling her at home. Somehow Margarita become a strength for the others, but Dr Shafford and I were aware that Margarita would benefit more by listening to herself rather than to the problems of others. It seemed to be in Margarita's nature that she wanted to help others but somehow could forget about herself. In 'My Lovely Blue Lady' she wrote 'how could she know I was crying inside all the time'. I felt the main issue was to find the tears that she so often talked about.

After the celebration event, we did a sound recording of her mother's life, from a text Margarita wrote at home. She wanted to do this in order to understand her mother better. Margarita said she could not understand why her mother was still visiting her as a ghost, and Margarita wanted to get rid of her as a ghost. She thought that by looking at their troubled relationship, she would be able to understand what had made her mother be so cruel to Margarita. We then edited the drawings into a moving sequence and added the sound, and it became an animation of her work. By concentrating on her mother's life, I was aware that Margarita could perhaps benefit from focusing more on her own being. I encouraged her to write about pleasant events in her life, and she wrote several short pieces about her life as a mother and wife, as a child being with her best friend, her Teddy and of her relationship with her younger brother, of whom she was very protective. Through writing about different aspects of her life, Margarita said 'life should be celebrated! Despite tragedy, there is life and life should be celebrated!'

During the summer, we made sound recordings of all her writings as she had an expressive voice.

Then one day in September, I visited her at home to work more with the writing. She read a poem to me that she had written when she was fourteen years old, in 1937. She said she had returned to the poem throughout her life, and had wanted to destroy it, but could not. She now felt strongly it was time to publish this poem. The poem is called 'A Body So Small' and portrays sexual abuse. Her stepfather abused her when she was nine and this experience shaped her life in many ways. She also felt it was necessary to tell this to other parents so other children could be helped.

That day we made a sound recording of the poem, she explained it and why she wrote it. We were recording the sound the first time she read it to me and I must admit I felt great sadness. I went quiet afterwards as I found it to be such a surprise and a very sad aspect of Margarita's life. The poem seemed to explain her other work, and I found the thread from the drawings to her writing, and why she was able to give so much to others. Margarita said 'the only thing you get from suffering is a deep understanding of others'.

A couple of weeks later, her health deteriorated quickly and she was admitted to the in-patient unit at the hospice. When I talked to her about the poem, and what to do with it, she said clearly she wanted to publish it on Rosetta Life's website. As she put it, 'it is the truth, and the truth should be told, although truth sometimes hurts'. As the poem portrays sexual abuse, Margarita was aware that it is painful but she also made clear that 'there is hope, look at me, I am 80-years-old and I have lived a happy life and you can get through to the other side'.

I felt that Margarita did not make herself a victim, but expressed how she had come full circle, having gained an understanding of what had happened. She said she did this by learning the reasons behind people's actions.

When I played the sound recording to her and showed the contextualisation I had written about 'A Body So Small' she said it was correct and presented in the way she wanted. As we spoke, Margarita was crying, but she said the crying gave her relief. I was reminded of the first time I met her when she told me she was not able to cry although she had so many tears inside. She told me her lovely blue lady was with her most of the time.

Although Margarita felt strongly that the poem should be published, she had not spoken with her sons about this and I was unsure if they knew about the abuse. As Rosetta Life artists, we work with individuals and their wishes are respected. In this case I felt that the sons should be informed. Margarita said she was going to tell them but as her illness progressed, she got increasingly tired and slept most of the time, so it would have been difficult to discuss the sound recording with her at that point. I spoke to staff at the

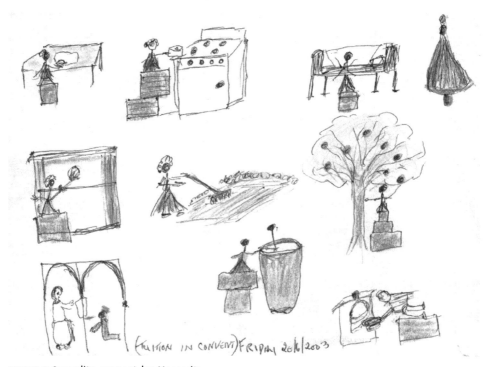

FIGURE 3 Carmelite convent by Margarita.

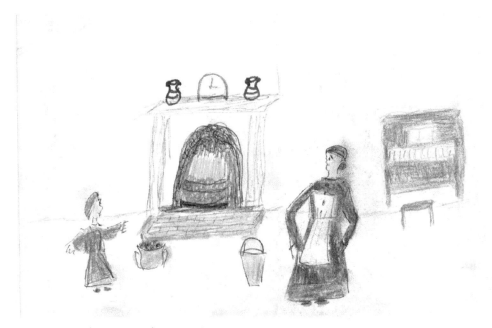

FIGURE 4 Carmelite convent by Margarita.

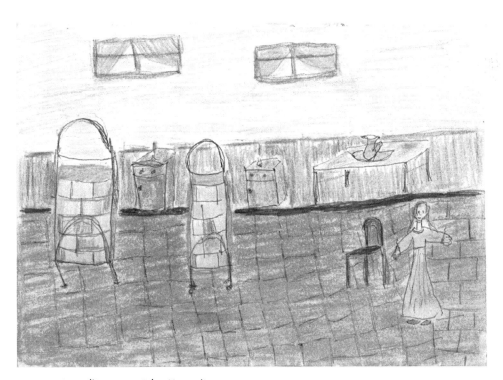

FIGURE 5 Carmelite convent by Margarita.

hospice about the situation and was encouraged to explain the situation to her sons. Staff were aware of issues that might arise and they could offer support to them if needed.

I talked to the sons about the poem and Margarita's wishes, and they told me they knew about the poem. I felt they had thought about it a lot, and that it was right to have informed them, although it was a difficult time. We decided to publish the poem and sound recordings.

Margarita died two days later.

I feel very privileged to have met Margarita. She gave me thoughts that I have reflected on several times, and her words will stay with me, as I know they will for several other people who were fortunate enough to meet her. Her calm presence and wisdom were enriching. Also, I am convinced that her presence is in her work, a legacy she left for others to gain enrichment and understanding in their lives.

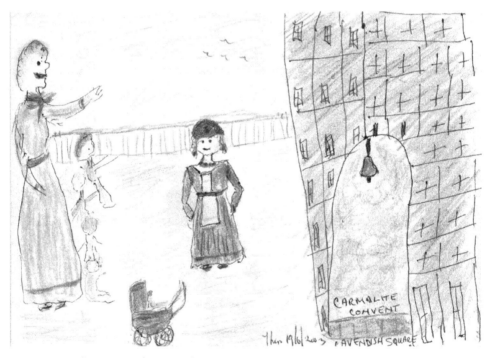

FIGURE 6 Carmelite convent by Margarita.

A Body So Small

Did you find delight in a body so small?
Did you thrill to the terror you made?
Did you stop her mouth so she couldn't call?
Did you enjoy your bodily raid?

Were you pleased the marks did not show?
Were you happy to get off scot free?
Were you proud of the dastardly blow?
Did you not hear the little ones plea?

'Please Daddie, don't do it again!'
You covered her mouth with your hand
And she cried silent tears for the pain
And the terror of no-man's land.

'I'll kill you if you ever tell
and you'll go to a home for sure'
She got off the bed and fell
In a despairing heap on the floor.

And now she is fully grown
A strange pretty girl said her friend
But a lover she never has known,
For her heart will not go to the end.

To a joy they say should be there;
For she sees only violence and rape
Where there should be loving care
And her life will never take shape

Are you still there Daddie dear?
Why you must be very proud
You gave your daughter a permanent tear.
It would be kinder to give her a shroud.

Margarita, written in 1937, 14 years old.

My Lovely Blue Lady

I am sitting in the moonlight, which is bathing me in beauty.
My heart is full of awe at the glory of the sky. It is very quiet and the night is caressing my face. I look around and there is my lovely blue lady coming towards me. She smiles and I think that she will pass me by, but no, she sits down beside me. I am aware of a beautiful perfume and the rustle of silk. I look away thinking she will vanish, but then I turn towards her, she is still there sitting radiantly in her beautiful blue dress, I can feel my heart banging and she takes my hand. I want to ask her if she will take me home with her, but I subconsciously know that is impossible. For some reason I feel desperately tired. She tells me not to worry and I try to relax and listen to what she is saying, but I cannot concentrate on the words only the lovely musical sounds, which comfort me. I ask her if she will show me how to live, because I seem to have lost my way and lack the discipline to put things right. She says walk one step at a time; until it becomes a habit, then move on to the next step. That seems very logical but I am not sure I will have enough self-discipline to follow her advice. She knows what I am thinking and promises to help me. I ask her what I can do for her and she tells me to go on loving her. I smile and so does she as I explain that I couldn't help loving her. She tells me I don't have to cry inside and I can cry every day if I want to. I wonder how she knows I cry inside all the time. I feel my lovely blue lady is a wise and kind spirit who knows me better than I know myself.

The Autumn Leaves Are Falling

The autumn leaves are falling, gently carpeting the world in gold. As I raise my eyes to the tall forest of trees the sunshine in glory through the dying leaves. I can hardly believe they are dying for their beauty is breathtaking. A slight breeze ruffles my hair and I relax into the woodland setting.

Nature herself is pointing the way to live and die. With joy and heavenly blue from spring bluebells, and happy dancing yellow daffodils, scarlet poppies and fields of waving corn to the gold of autumn.

Shades of night are falling as I make my way homeward, the leaves crunching under my feet and a feeling of peace in my heart.

How can I ever thank the great creator for the gift of such beauty, and how many lives will it take before all the messages handed down in love can be understood?

Margarita

Margarita

Dr Elizabeth Shafford

Margarita was diagnosed with carcinoma of the left breast in 1999 at the age of 76. The tumour was oestrogen and progesterone positive and so she was treated with Tamoxifen to which she had a good response but Margarita requested to discontinue this treatment as she felt that it was making her forgetful. In December 2000 she was changed to Arimidex to which she again had a good response but Margarita stopped this treatment in October 2002, because of hot flushes, unbeknown to her oncologist. In November 2002 she developed a small break in the skin over the tumour, which was then 1.5 x 2 cm. It was not until June 2003 that Margarita admitted that she was no longer taking hormone therapy and Megestrol Acetate was commenced. By that time the tumour measured 5 x 3 cm.

Her past medical history is relevant in that she had a major road traffic accident in her 20s when she was run over by a 10 ton lorry resulting in a fractured pelvis and crushed legs. She was in plaster for 6 months and in hospital for 1 year.

She was registered disabled in 1985.

Some of her pain and her poor mobility was related to this accident and not her cancer. She also had macular degeneration which affected her ability to read and write, which was a source of frustration.

At the time of her first attendance at day care in July 2003 Margarita's main problems were pain in her left shoulder, emotional distress and low self-worth.

She was an obese lady with poor mobility who used a wheelchair in day care to get from A to B. Transferring to the examination couch was quite an ordeal as a consequence of her previous RTA.

The fungating area in the left breast was submammary and measured 2 × 1cm. There was no odour and a minimal discharge.

During Margarita's first visit to day care it became evident that there were many events in her past that she was struggling to understand and come to terms with. These issues were freely expressed in response to enquiries about her family, how she felt that she was coping with her illness, and whether she was sustained by a religious faith or spiritual belief.

She had a fear that she was suffering from dementia because she was experiencing recurring thoughts about her mother. She could not understand why these thoughts were intruding on her at this time as her mother had been dead for about 15 years. I suggested that because of her illness she was less active which allowed these unwelcomed thoughts, which had probably previously been subconscious, to reach her consciousness. I think the fear of dementia was related to the fact that she had nursed her husband who died from lead poisoning.

Margarita was an illegitimate child born whilst her mother's husband was away from home serving in the army. She never met her father and her mother never told her anything about him. She was seriously ill as a baby and was not expected to survive. From the age of 4–9 years she was sent away from home to live with someone that she did not know. When she returned home at the age of 9 her stepfather started to sexually abuse her.

In her mid 20s Margarita had a miscarriage – soon after that she married a man 23 years her senior who had been a 'father figure' for many years.

Margarita had worked as an English teacher in a London stage school and taught a number of now famous actors who continued to keep in touch with her but she did not see this as any sort of achievement and had very low self-worth.

Margarita lived with her youngest son, although they had their own flats in the same house. She was very concerned about the demands that she was putting on this son who worked as a music teacher giving lessons in schools and at home, and she did all that she could to maintain her independence.

Margarita was brought up a Roman Catholic but at one time after she was married she became involved with Jehovah's Witnesses for several years. She expressed the concern that although she could pray for others she was unable to pray for herself.

Margarita was an intelligent woman and she was aware that by discontinuing her hormone treatment without telling anyone she could well have influenced the course of her disease. She had a concern that her action might influence the way that she would be treated.

She was quite distressed by the presence of the fungating wound in her breast. Although there was no associated odour and only a very slight discharge, the fact that it needed dressing was a constant reminder of her disease and its progression.

Margarita was very keen to talk. If given the opportunity she would monopolise whoever was willing to listen. Although she frequently told us that we must tell her to 'shut up' I don't think any member of staff felt comfortable doing this as she had so much that she needed to share.

Margarita was reluctant to complain of pain perhaps because she had experienced pain for many years as a result of the RTA. She would quite easily get off the subject of her physical symptoms and talk about the painful events in the past. I found that with me she would often go over the same ground, but the Rosetta Life artist in residence was more skilful in helping Margarita to explore these feelings and move forward.

I also found it difficult to gauge Margarita's awareness of her illness as in the same breath she would talk about dying and then say that she expected me to enable her to live to 100 so that she would outlive her mother who died at the age of 96.

On her initial presentation in day care the psychosocial issues were felt to be at least as, if not more, important than the physical symptoms. Margarita was offered the opportunity to speak with the chaplain, as she was felt to be suffering some spiritual distress relating to her inability to pray for herself, and also, what she described as, the intrusion of her mother into her life.

She was also introduced to the Rosetta Life – artist in residence Heidi and with her help, through a process of drawings and writings, began to reach an understanding of her mother's life and to understand better her own feeling of abandonment.

Margarita was very reluctant to take any tablets for pain. At the time of first attendance at day care she was only taking paracetamol which was not controlling her shoulder pain. She was given Co-codamol 8/500 which she would only take on an as needed basis.

In August 2003 she complained of a dull aching pain in her left lower chest which was worse on deep breathing and movement. She was tender over the lower ribs anteriorly.

A chest X-ray was performed looking for bone metastases. Although no bony disease was identified diclofenac was thought to be an appropriate analgesic in view of the local tenderness. Diclofenac SR 75mg b.d. and lansoprazole was commenced but this caused nausea and vomiting and so was discontinued.

The left sided chest pain continued and was associated with left sided abdominal pain and abdominal distension. Examination was suggestive of ascites.

An abdominal ultrasound was perfomed to confirm the presence of ascites as this patient was not known to have intra abdominal disease. Ascites was confirmed but the liver was small and no tumour masses were identified. Her analgesics were changed to Co-codamol 30/500 which she finally agreed to take regularly, with some improvement in her pain. She was admitted to the in-patient unit for paracentesis and 3.5 litres of fluid were drained and examination of the fluid showed it to be an exudate.

Paracentesis relieved the abdominal distension but Margarita continued to be in pain in spite of regular Co-codamol. She was initially very reluctant to change to morphine but we gradually gained her trust and she agreed to a trial of morphine. As this was effective and because of her reluctance to take tablets she was changed to a Fentanyl patch initially 25mcg/24 hours. She was experiencing nausea at this time thought to be related to the ascites but she declined any antiemetics. She was also reluctant to take laxatives because of her difficulty in getting to the toilet when at home, because of her poor mobility. Spironolactone was started with the aim of preventing/delaying reaccumulation of ascites.

At the end of August she was reviewed by her oncologist and Anastrazole was added to her hormone treatment and she was also started on Domperidone for nausea.

Margarita continued to attend day care on a weekly basis and spent time with Heidi at each visit. Her pain was not completely controlled but she was reluctant to take morphine for breakthrough pain. Her abdomen was distended but this was thought to be mainly gaseous distension rather than ascites. Peppermint water was suggested for relief of wind and Margarita agreed to a trial of Celicoxib for her pain which was thought to be due to presumed peritoneal disease.

At the end of September her condition deteriorated with anorexia, dysphagia, nausea and vomiting, loss of weight, diarrhoea and faecal incontinence, and worsening mobility and she was again admitted to the in-patient unit. On admission she was commenced on a syringe driver with metoclopromide to control her nausea and vomiting which was thought to be due to squashed stomach syndrome caused by her ascites. This markedly improved but did not control her nausea so Haloperidol was later added with good effect. The diarrhoea and faecal incontinence was thought to be due to constipation with overflow. An abdominal X-ray was done at this point as it was difficult to palpate the abdomen because of ascites. This showed faecal loading and rectal measures were started but with little improvement in Margarita's symptoms. Because of continuing deterioration rectal intervention was stopped, with cessation of faecal oozing.

Dysphagia was thought to be due to oral and oesophageal candidias. Margarita had been on Fluconazole for 2 weeks because of oral candida, so this was changed to Itraconazole solution. However as her condition deteriorated she became unable to take any oral medications.

Margarita died peacefully 2 weeks after her admission with her sons by her side.

When Margarita was in day care there was little contact with the family. However when Margarita was in the in-patient unit there was the opportunity to speak with both her sons and the daughter-in-law and granddaughter.

In the initial weeks of Margarita's involvement with the hospice I thought that she and her youngest son, were trying to protect each other and I felt that they were not being open with each other. After the paracentesis Margarita was insistent that she should get out of bed and get dressed otherwise her sons would think that she was really ill. However she did not keep up this pretence during the final weeks of her illness.

Margarita's eldest son and his family live in Germany. Margarita insisted that her granddaughter, who had come over from Germany to see her, returned to take up her place at music college. This caused some distress to her granddaughter and her daughter-in-law as they both felt guilty about leaving when they knew that they would not see Margarita alive again. Some time was spent trying to support them in a decision that they didn't want to make.

I found Margarita a fascinating albeit time consuming patient to deal with. She had quite a story to tell and through listening to her it became evident how much her childhood experiences continued to influence her. In spite of all that she achieved as an English teacher in a stage school and as a wife, mother and grandmother, she had no self-worth because she was made to feel of no significance as a child.

Certainly when she first came to the hospice these issues were of more importance to her than her physical symptoms.

Margarita had lived with the consequences of her childhood experiences all of her life. Only when she became physically less active as a result of her illness did she allow these issues to reach her consciousness. She was a troubled lady when she arrived in day care but over the ensuing weeks chiefly through her work with Rosetta Life but also with the support of the chaplain and medical and nursing staff she was able to find peace.

I found it a real privilege to get to know Margarita during the last few months of her life, and I am sure that I will remember her for a long time to come. She has certainly deepened my understanding of the importance of dealing with psychosocial issues for the wellbeing of a patient. Margarita was an easy patient to help in that she was quite open and volunteered a great deal of information.

Concentrating solely on her physical symptoms would not have dealt with these underlying issues and demonstrates the importance of holistic care.

Heidi Morstang is an artist specialising in photography and the moving image. Between January 2003 and July 2004 she worked part time as a Rosetta Life artist at St Luke's Hospice, Basildon and at St Margaret's Hospice, Taunton, where she worked mainly with video. Heidi photographed her father during his illness of skin cancer, documenting his changing appearance during his last months. This resulted in a touring exhibition in Scandinavia in collaboration with the Norwegian Cancer Organisation.

Dr Elizabeth Shafford has worked in child health and paediatrics with twenty years' experience in the field of paediatric oncology running clinics for teenagers and young adults. After time spent at Belgrave Children's Hospital, Kings College and Great Ormond Street, she moved to work part time at St Luke's Hospice, Basildon, where she works primarily in Day Care.

CHAPTER 3

A guide to living with cancer according to PG Wodehouse

Katherine Vaughan-Williams

A playscript performed by Gary Stevens at Hampstead Theatre, London in 2003.

Gary Stevens presented Katherine Vaughan-Williams' profoundly moving monologue about the tumours that came to stay – in her own body. This work was developed in partnership with Rosetta Life who produced the final theatre work that was first performed at Hampstead Theatre in July 2003.

Imagine if you will a village hall entertainment. Assorted corn chandlers and seed merchants are settling down into a soothing reverie coincident with arriving half-way through the evening's offering's. There is a frowst in here you could cut with a knife. The hesitant and inexperienced speaker's reluctance to appear is dealt with by the decisive shove in the small of the back by an unseen hand. He shambles on to a chorus of assorted shuffles and coughs and announces:

Have you ever been in the curious position of seeing your native bearer torn limb from limb by hungry tigers, just after you yourself have safely shinned up a tree and pulled it up after you? Well, what do you experience? A silent prayerful relief that it is him, not you, who is getting it properly in the neck, followed by a short head with due regret at seeing a fellow sufferer disappearing down the pan.

(Caption) ROCKY III: The Lump Returns

I first knew I was in for a rough ride when I saw the scans. The lumps turned up in my body unannounced, without so much as a by your leave, let alone a formal invitation, and in fact they were not at all the sort of character you would invite within miles of your person, given the choice, which I wasn't. It was like coming home from an unremarkable few days break on the South Coast to discover that, unbeknown to you, a large pink blighter with a beer gut, an objectionable leer and a gang of shifty-looking hangers on had insinuated themselves into every one of your holiday snaps. They were back. With their hair in a braid.

I don't know how they had got in but I was jolly well resolved that they were not going to stay there picnicking at my expense any longer. I could clearly discern the image of a whacking big tumour, lying on the floor and staring up at me in rather an austere manner, as if it wanted a written explanation and apology. There was something about the thing's expression that absolutely chilled me and I withdrew on tip-toe and shut the door.

After a couple of much needed swift ones, courtesy of the barman at the Bollinger, I returned home refreshed and revived.

'What became of the tumour, Jeeves?' I said.

'It is in your liver, sir.'

'What!'

'Yes, sir.'

'In my liver?'

'Yes sir. I summoned a medical man who gave it as his opinion that the tumour should remain for the time being in situ.'

'You mean the blighter is on the premises for an indefinite visit?'

'Yes sir.'

I found the tumour lying in my upper right lobe, draped in a suit of my heliotrope pyjamas, smoking one of my cigarettes and reading a detective story. It waved the cigarette at me in what I considered a dashed patronizing manner.

'Ah, Wooster!' It said.

'Not so much of the Ah Wooster,' I replied brusquely, 'How soon can you be removed?'

'Oh, in about six months or so, I fancy.'

'Six months!'

'Possibly. For the moment the doctor insists on perfect quiet and repose. So, forgive me, old man, for asking you not to raise your voice or get yourself worked up in any way. A Buddha-like hushed whisper is the stuff to give us tumours.'

Well, I wasn't going to stand around and listen to bilge about serenity and calm, culled from the problem pages of dubious magazines. I remained firmly incandescent. 'Are you sure you can't be removed?'

'Quite. The doctor said so.'

'I think we ought to get a second opinion.'

'Useless, my dear fellow. He was most emphatic and evidently a man who knew his job. Please don't worry about my not being comfortable here. I shall be quite all right. I like your liver. And now, returning to the issue in hand. My sister will be arriving tomorrow and will naturally want to stay. I am her favourite brother.'

'You are?'

'I am.'

'How many of you are there?'

'Six.'

'And you are her favourite brother?'

A girl, I felt of unnatural, not to say morbid tastes.

'As a matter of fact, old thing, when I say six, I should have mentioned earlier that there's a fairly sporting chance that my aunt and a number of relatives, small and large, have arrived in the interim and well, to look the thing in the face, I'm afraid, that we have rather spread ourselves...'

It looked anything but sorry, in fact it looked dashed pleased with itself that some other poor sucker was being driven to the wall.

It took a refreshing drag of one of my best Turkish that I reserve for my private use and went on, 'it's quite probable that you'll find the gang scattered around the place and parked in various nooks and crannies. In fact a couple of them are, what you might call, near neighbours and have fixed themselves up in your lymph nodes. All rather cosy and jolly I'm sure you'll agree.'

I did not agree, and stomped off in what you might call a marked manner.

'Jeeves,' I said, 'This tumour appears to be a fixture.'

'Yes, sir.'

'Or should I say tumours. It appears that two of them are lurking in my personal lymph nodes, which I require for other and, I might add, more fitting uses. And tomorrow we shall have his sister in our midst.'

'What is my body, Liberty Hall? It appears to be open season for cancer, dash it.'

He assumed the sober expression of a concerned tomato.

'I can well appreciate your feelings, sir.'

'That's all very well,' I said moodily smashing a figurine of a well-known oncologist against the chimney-breast, 'but have you got any suggestions?'

'I must confess that the situation does seem somewhat intractable, sir. I have formulated a solution which however, I'm not sure will meet wholly with your approval. I fancy we may find a way to remove the incumbents, with difficulty, but only after you have been through a rather trying experience. There is someone we may call on to offer aid, but I fear he might well leave you a mere shadow of your former self.'

'I can take some roughs with some smooths, as Anatole, would have it. Better a mere shadow, Jeeves ...'

'In that case, sir, I feel we have no alternative but to call on the somewhat dubious services of Baxter Bottle.'

30 second Charleston
(*Caption*) THIS IS NOT GOING TO HURT ME AS MUCH AS IT HURTS YOU

When you look at it in the face, chemotherapy is quite simply a poison, and a poison which a more-than-usually bilious Crippen would have hesitated to administer to his least favourite bride. Thus it is somewhat curious that within hospitals, chemotherapy is treated with a kind of awed reverence normally associated with chef Anatole's peerless cuisine at Brinkley Court, Gloucestershire.

The great thing with chemotherapy is to have it 'fresh'. So fresh that the most starched of matrons coo like young mothers over its dew-like bloom. Next, it must be so expensive that hardened financiers stop in their tracks and swing back on their heels with a startled whistle of admiration. Luckily for us, in re. this last characteristic Messers. Bayer, Smith Kline-Glaxo and their colleagues are happy to oblige. Before the order for chemotherapy can be accepted by the kitchen, however, the patient has to undergo minute examination to make sure that he is up to the mark. A lackadaisical outlook, particularly by white blood cells, will be taken amiss. Any absence of enthusiasm on their part and you will find that your consultant has all the politesse of a short-tempered maitre d', and you will be out on your ear before you can say 'sylphides a la crème'.

If the all clear is given, then follows a rather longer than usual stage wait. To clarify: this is a wait which makes an ordinary common or garden wait look like a mere flicker in the eyebrow of recorded time. While waiting for chemotherapy, people have been known to meet, fall in love, get married and fall out over which parent-in-law they will fob the children off on at Christmas; international relations between superpowers have deteriorated, exploded and got all pally again.

As you drank in the twilight waiting room that is chemotherapy limbo, you will notice a baldish, wanish looking chap sidle up to you. That, of course, in no way distinguishes him from the hoardes of other baldish, wanish looking blokes propped up in various corners, who are only to be expected given the exclusive constitution of the club into which you have just been accepted. This one, however, has a faintly jaunty, sporting aspect. He stuffs a well-used bit of card in your shirt pocket. To hand it back with a look of appropriate hauteur is with you the work of a moment, at which point the chap mutters out of the corner of his mouth,

'Well, are you in or what?'

'What?'

'Listen, old horse, do you feel in want of a sporting flutter.'

'You interest me strangely. Proceed.'

'Well, you know how much chemo there is round here.'

'The thing hadn't escaped my notice.'

'There are about half-a-dozen different sorts, and each chemo is the ewe lamb of a consultant, and each consultant has got its patient. Today we're running off the great chemo handicap. I'm making the book. Each chemo is to be clocked by a reliable steward of the course and the one that takes longest to get attached, wins.'

'Yes, but why the card?'

'Why you utter chump, it gives the handicaps and current odds on each starter chemo. Take a careful look at it: it gives you the thing in a nutshell.'

On the race card I read the following words:

Chemo handicap
Runners and Betting
Probable starters:
Oxaliplatin (Dr Agatha Spenser-Gregson): Scratch
Oxaliplatin plus 5FU (Sir Roderick Glossop (seconded from psychiatry)): Scratch
Irinotecan (Dr Montgomery Bodkin): Receives 2 hours and forty minutes.
5FU (Dr Hilda Gudgeon): Receives 4 hours and forty minutes.
Ironetcan plus 5FU (Prof. E Jimpson-Murgatgroyd): receives 5 hours
The above have arrived:
Prices: 5–2 Spenser-Gregson, Glossop; 3–1 Bodkin; 6–1 Gudgeon, Jimpson-Murgatroyd

Now, tell me, has anything struck you yet about that card? No? It's obviously a sitter for 5FU. 5FU for those not in the know, is the snappy nickname for a quite unpronounceable concoction which, it is claimed, is the Gold Standard for chemotherapy. In other words it is the acronym for something the medical profession have been fobbing punters off with for the best part of five decades, when they can't think of anything better to do. For Gold Standard here read poor relation: 5FU has the status of the soda in a whisky and s – and is about as effective – while the chemotherapy heavy mob are the equivalent of Glenmorangie and The Macallan. Oncologists are happy to swing the 5FU siphon at the drop of a needle. 5FU is cheap, it's abundant, it comes out of the lab quicker than a jackrabbit and it has just earned you 120 smackeroonies at 6–1.

And so the chemotherapy emerges, accompanied by the smiles of the nursing staff, a blast of the Toreadors chorus from the 4th act of Carmen and sporting what appears to be a diminutive tuxedo in a dressy peacock blue.

Beneath its external garb the chemotherapy is enshrined within a pint sized bottle, which bears the sinister legend 'Baxter B. ref.c1009'. This Baxter is a shifty looking character; a chap who makes a profession of latching himself via an unfeasibly long tube onto other people's bodies. The general idea is to shove the stuff straight into your bloodstream, so bypassing the usual channels. The bottle's outlook on life is grim. He is not one of those fun loving bits of medical equipment, who sport a multi coloured party hat and accompanying whoopee whistle and who consider the day ill-spent until they have turned a few cartwheels and retired to universal applause. He is a serious bloke, steeped to the gills with moral purpose. There is this to say in his favour, though, Baxter is efficient. At his bugle call, squatting tumours up sticks and canter off into the sunset, unlamented by one and all.

You will have spotted the downside of course. In rendering the body thoroughly unfit for inhabitation, the zealous activities of the Baxter Bottle would have the unavoidable knock-on effect of turning that pleasant and restful abode into a realm of terror, trembling and gnashing of teeth.

But, despite this obvious disadvantage, he wears the inexplicably self-satisfied air of a man getting ready to receive the thanks of the nation, tapping at your chest the while as if to suggest that you are a lucky chap to have Baxter Bottles working day and night in your interests. He has it firmly rooted in his mind that he is the popular hero, beloved of all - little knowing that your favourite reading would be the legend 'Baxter. B. ref c1009' on a tombstone. Rather saddening the whole thing.

30 second Charleston: 'Singing in the Rain'
(*Caption*) III. YES MEN AND VICE YESSERS

It is not easy to explain to the lay mind the extremely intricate ramifications of a Major London Teaching Hospital. Scanning the roster of those doctors I have been embroiled with in my time we come across some tough babies. Starting at the top: The Professor. He has a pair of shaggy eyebrows that give his eyes a piercing outlook, which is not at all the sort of thing a fellow wants to encounter when tethered to a drip, let alone attached to a catheter and on an empty stomach. He is fairly tall and fairly broad and has the most enormous head with practically no hair on it, thereby showing what a rotten thing it is to let your brain develop too much.

The Professor is generally spotted by the ordinary punter accompanied with a gang of gawping hangers-on clustering round his bed. At this point it should be noted that attempts to propitiate or establish a friendly rapport by hailing him with the words, Hi, prof, take a pew, are of little or no efficacy.

The experienced medical observer will learn in time to distinguish the various members of the Professor's accompanying crew of assorted limpets. They consist of Senior Yes Men, Second Yes Men, Vice Yessers, Junior Yes Men and Nodders. Putting it as briefly as possible for the lay mind, a Nodder is something like a Yes Man, only lower on the social scale. A Yes person's duty is to attend case conferences and say, 'Yes'. A Nodder's, as the name implies, is to nod.

Gathered round the bed on which the specimen under examination lies prone, the Professor throws out some statement of opinion, and looks about him expectantly. This is the cue for the senior Yes Man, or consultant, to say 'yes'. He is followed, in order of precedence, by the second Yes Man or Senior Registrar, as he is sometimes called, Vice-Yesser or Registrar and the junior Yes Man or Houseman. Only when all the Yes Men have yessed do the Nodders begin to function.

They nod. True, it may not sound like much of a job. Not very exalted. However, there is also a class of untouchables who are known as Nodders' assistants or junior doctors.

The Nodder's assistant or Junior Doctor is to be found on the outskirts of the charmed bed circle. Not only is he never to be seen oscillating the bean, but he has in addition the general outlook and appearance of one stuffed by a half-hearted taxidermist. He will be wearing a suit into which he has been poured at 3 o'clock the previous afternoon, and habitually be seen staring into the middle distance as if in a sort of miasma or trance.

When his eye is caught he will blush becomingly and turn his head away, like a shy, wild rose caught in a sudden, fragrant breeze.

It is Easter weekend and a desert wind had blown in through the corridors of the hospital. Every other doctor had made a break for the open spaces. It was like one of the great race movements that you read about. Only two Nodders assistants remained in situ to carry on the work of 126 assorted Nodders, junior Yes Men, Vice Yessers, second Yes Men, senior Yes Men and indeed the Professor himself.

Left in the hands of a Nodder's assistant the patients anticipate an educational few days attempting communication with one who, for all signs of intelligent life he had previously exhibited, might be deemed to have gone AWOL from a fishmonger's slab.

The first day, the patient receives a nasty shock. Not only had the Nodder's assistant shed the suit and is now sporting a rugby shirt in an especially loathsome shade of mustard yellow, the beginnings of a smirk and has successfully negotiated his way to the patient's bedside. There the Nodder's assistant contributes to his already not inconsiderable trauma by addressing the patient by name. It is thus established beyond all reasonable doubt that his mouth though undeniably cod-like, can nevertheless speak and perform rudimentary reading.

The second day, a further sartorial sensation takes place as the Nodder's assistant dons combat fatigues and trainers.

Despite the fact that the patient is unable to proffer an opinion due to an assortment of ten tubes emerging from orifices, natural and man-made, the Junior Doctor makes himself at home on his bed while confiding in him in an offensively pally manner that Senior Staff Nurse Bassett really is the business. The third day, the transformation is accomplished. A new man, he is clad in flip-flops, singlet and footer bags and he has clearly got it right up his nose.

To eliminate your De Gramond chemotherapy regime with a single imperious gesture and substitute a super-intensive daily course of Taliban in combination with the experimental drug Vomitzidon, is with him the work of a moment.

Unfortunately, it is at that same moment that the Professor picks to sneak back early. The Nodder's assistant emits a sharp gurgle and shies like a startled mustang. He has retreated to the wall and to seem, as far as the patient can gather, to be trying to get through it. But not before the Prof has been able to decipher amongst the Nodder's assistants inarticulate gibberings something about De Gramond's Approved Chemo-Therapy Regime that does not bear repetition.

The patient wonders silently what this has been. Evidently something red hot, for it is clear that it still rankles like a boil on the back of the neck. The Professor's fists, he sees, are clenched and he has started to tap his foot on the ground - sure indication that the amour-propre is fed to the eye-teeth. He is one of those oncologists who look upon De Gramond's Approved Regime as a sort of personal buddy and receive with an ill grace cracks at its expense.

The patient feels like a man who, stooping to pluck a nosegay of wild flowers on a railway line, is unexpectedly hit in the small of the back by the Cornish Express. He lies, superfluous behind a stained curtain and listens to the animal cries of a distinguished Professor as he attempts to turn a Junior Doctor inside out and make him swallow himself.

And he becomes convinced that all this must be that Collapse of Civilisation of which he has so often spoken with such eloquence at his local Rotary Club Meetings.

30 second Charleston: 'The Black Bottom'

After the thing is all over, when peril has ceased to loom and happy endings have been distributed in heaping handfuls and we are driving home with our hats on the side of our heads, I confess to Jeeves that there were moments during the recent proceedings when I came very near to despair.

'Within a toucher, Jeeves.'

'Unquestionably, affairs had developed a certain menacing trend.'

'I couldn't see a ray of hope. It looked to me as if the blue bird had thrown in the towel and formally ceased to function. And yet here we are, all boomps-a-daisy. There's an expression on the tip of my tongue that seems to me to sum the whole thing up. Or rather, when I say an expression, I mean a saying. A wheeze. A gag. Something about Joy doing something.'

'Joy cometh in the morning, sir?'

'That's the baby. Not one of your things, is it?'

'No, sir.'

'Well, it's dashed good,' I said.

Katherine Vaughan-Williams and PG Wodehouse

Nicholas Pope, June 2004

The generative ideas for this piece were born before Kath was ill and when she was still working at Southbank University. The time between tutorials would often be spent with her musing with myself and Jeremy Melvin on the fact that Wodehouse had something to offer in response to any human condition, however distressing. The realisation was that his writing could be experienced as medicine in the form of words. When Kath contracted cancer, the project took on a very serious sense of urgency. That this piece was written polished and performed towards the very end of her life is a remarkable testament to her ability to radiate light, humour and positivity whatever her circumstances. What lies behind the writing is extremely profound – it is an emphatic confirmation of the redemptive power of words if assembled with infinite care and their ability to provide a gateway to that which lies beyond our material and physical existence – the realm of pure imagination. Kath conceived of another project to follow this one, the title of which could be seen as the embodiment of the gesture of her life: it was to be called the PG Wodehouse Guide to Love.

Katherine Vaughan-Williams was an influential architectural historian and writer. She adored 1960s radio comedy and PG Wodehouse who inspired this work. Katherine died in September 2003.

Gary Stevens developed the work for performance. He is a visual artist who has worked in the field of live performance from a background of installation and film since 1984.

CHAPTER 4

Arts in palliative care: the Prince and Princess of Wales Hospice

Marielle Macleman

The Prince and Princess of Wales Hospice is situated in four adjacent townhouses in the centre of Glasgow, a city with diverse social demographics and a high rate of cancer. Providing clinical, emotional, social and spiritual care for patients who have a progressive, life-threatening illness, the hospice has a conventional medical model. The introduction of an innovative arts project in 2003 reflected a commitment to develop new therapeutic initiatives and to investigate the potential of a needs-led approach. Arts in Palliative Care provided cultural and creative opportunities that would otherwise be inaccessible to patients. Initiating from a twelve-week pilot proposed by Glasgow City Council and established arts organisation Art in Hospital, it filled a gap in arts provision within palliative care in Glasgow, drawing on the combined experience of participants, healthcare and arts professionals, and local authority cultural and leisure services. The project provided an important bridge between two care models in the redesign of day services, and responding to patient feedback, the hospice facilitated its continuation and integration to a multidisciplinary referral procedure and documentation. The following accounts reveal the pivotal role of participants in shaping the arts project and subsequent developments in hospice facilities, staff education and recruitment. A day services patient and participant of the arts project, John Lieser recounts his personal journey, illustrating the value of user involvement for the participant and hospice alike.

In this chapter I have collaborated with a service user, John. I, working as artist co-ordinator of arts in palliative care, elaborate on the positive and negative implications of the project's development from an organisational perspective and John tells the story from the perspective of a patient. Ultimately, each of us cite the potential of art to develop a voice, and to provide a platform for that voice to be heard.

John's journey: finding a voice

I've been coming to the hospice for about four and a half years. A consultant gave me a matter of weeks to live and that was a wee bit on the low side of my life. When I first walked through the door I expected to see people in wheelchairs and on stretchers, people dying here and dying there. That was my first reaction and I really didn't want to become one of the statistics. I was very low.

After about an hour, I realised that the atmosphere, the people and the way the place was run was really something else. That lifted my morale a good bit. Even after an hour. People were so pleasant and they couldn't do enough for me. That really struck me as a positive step in my life, after being diagnosed and told the bad news.

The day unit had a pool table, dominoes and a few other wee things like bingo, the things that you would get in your normal life, which was really good for me. It was 2001 and I had only been there for about six months when a pilot art project started. I wasn't really interested in art. Even when the lady asked me if I would like to try something and I said I wasn't really into that sort of thing. I had been denied it at school, so I didn't feel I would have been any good at it, but the artist gently persuaded me over a number of days to try it.

She gave me a piece of white paper and watercolours. She asked me if I was sure that I didn't do any art at school, and I said no, I didn't do any art at school. I'll always remember that my first painting was of a Russian lady, just a portrait of her that I copied from the book. I thought it was absolutely rubbish! It looked as if a young child had done it. That's how I felt. I was a wee bit embarrassed about it in fact, because I thought it was that bad, but she saw something in it that I didn't. She asked me twice, was I sure that I didn't get art at school and I said no, because I'd never even tried drawing with a pencil

I stuck with the art and they really gave me a lot of encouragement. After a few weeks I realised, myself, that this is not a bad thing and this is really keeping me away from my illness. For the time I was sitting painting, I forgot all about my illness. It really took me to a new depth within myself. I could get lost in this painting and forgot about everything that felt bad to me at that time. It was then I realised that other patients could maybe get the same benefit from it that I did. And they did.

I went over to the other patients and they kept saying 'I can't, I can't' and I told them that neither could I, but I sat down and I realised that there is something there. Then I sold my first painting at the Glasgow Art Fair. That was tremendous. From being a 'zero' at art, to selling a painting was really great. Everyone realised that this was a great thing. I started taking my camcorder in to film the workshops and show everyone how their painting looked on the hospice TV. This was of great excitement to the other patients. It got everyone involved in that way.

After about four months the funds dried up. I bought myself an easel, brushes and paints. I paint at the edge of my garage. You get a lot of people interested as they're passing by. I find that really good. But we really missed the art. Every time the Chief Executive came down to see us I was 'heckling', if you like. Every time a dignitary came in I'd ask if they had any funding – like when the Scottish Secretary for Health visited. I wasn't letting a thing get by me on that! Hospice staff would always come to get my view. They didn't prompt me but they'd say, 'this is such and such John', and they knew I was rambling on about the funding, so they knew what was coming. It wasn't only me. It was every artist involved that wanted the art class back. Everyone needed this art back. They were getting the same thing as I was – they were forgetting about their illness.

I was told there wasn't any room for art. I had to make quite an effort to bring the art project back but, again, it helped me with my illness. Having that on my mind gave me a goal to achieve. It could be the last thing I ever did properly in my life. Fortunately, I'm a lot better now. We kept on at it. It took well over a year and eventually the Chief Executive said 'we've got good news and bad news'. 'We've got the funding but we haven't got a place'. So again, we said 'well, if you've got the funding, we'll get the place' and eventually they gave us a wee room next door.

I was quite deeply involved in setting up the project when it returned. The hospice invited us to pick the artists. This felt brilliant. It gave us some respect back and said to us that 'we are important people in here'. It gave me a new lease of life. I wasn't anxious about this as, before I came to the hospice, I was involved in committees and what have you, so I was a wee bit experienced in that side of things. I had to give these up because of ill health, so involvement in the recruitment process somehow made up for that. However, it was a totally different thing from employing someone to just do a job.

We were given the six names, six people turned up. They were prompt and they all gave a really good account of themselves but Marielle and her partner were really good. They stood out from the rest. We didn't want just anybody in here. 'Anybody' wouldn't have suited us. We needed someone who would not just look on it as a nine to five job, but someone dedicated to making sure that we got the best out of the art as possible. I mean, the girl comes in three days a week but she'd come in on a Friday, which is not our dedicated art day, to see if we wanted any paints, asking if the brushes we had were ok. We thought that this was absolutely fantastic, that the girl really cares for us. I think it's more important than artistic abilities. You could be a great artist but if you don't have that feeling about the person, then it's no use.

It wouldn't have been right for someone to just come in and say 'This is your new artist'. We would have felt left out of things. Being involved was marvellous because I think that, as people with cancer, we've got a better ability to perceive things about people who are going to be working with patients with the illness. I think we're able to recognise any deficiency.

I think it's important that others learn from somebody that lives with cancer, because they're talking from experience. My experience when I was first diagnosed was that people were frightened to talk to me. The word 'hospice' puts terror into people. They would cross the street before having a word with you. You begin to feel it's infectious or something. They don't want to ask how you're doing in case you break down and cry or become abusive towards them. It's important for nurses and doctors to hear that from you.

The actual patient knows more about the cancer. Doctors and nurses know how to treat you, but they don't know what it is to have cancer. They just don't know what's in your mind. This is the big thing. Even the professors and the like, they just say 'we'll give you this' and 'we'll give you that' but they never think of how you're feeling with the scars left behind. The scars of radiotherapy, when you get the top load of 34 doses. It leaves you in a terrible position even years after, you still get bother swallowing. Then again, you've got to acknowledge when they say 'you're here today'. That's an important thing you've got to remember as well, although you went through all that, you're here today and you wouldn't be here today if you didn't get treatment.

After the art project was established, I was invited to the Southern General Hospital to talk about my experiences to a group of nurses. I was told there was going to be a few people there, but I was astonished to find that there was 96 people there and that really drew my breath back a wee bit. My biggest fear was that, because treatment had meant I couldn't pronounce my words, they wouldn't understand what I was going on about. I wanted them to understand everything I wanted to say about the illness, the hospice and everyone I've been involved with. Before I went I had prepared a speech with help from the Creative Writer in Residence, but when you make a speech there's always something more you want to tell or something compacted into your memory. But I kept to the script. I told them just like it was. That again helped get through a bad part of my life. It really helped me get it off my chest. I was so embarrassed with the applause I got, I wanted to get up and run out the door!

There's thousands of cancer patients who would have said the same but they didn't have the opportunity. Patients say, 'I wish I could say something'. I personally asked for a suggestion box in the hospice so that we can keep the patients involved and so that it wouldn't be demeaning asking 'can I have this?' and 'can I have that?' A lot of things have come forth. If the hospice had changed anything, we'd ask them to change it back. It's good that we have a direct line to whoever is to do things. I've had word back on things. They actually post a letter to your house if you give them your name and address. It's good because at least you're getting listened to.

It's not big things, just wee things we would like to change. I would love a cup of tea after my lunch. I'd love to be taken away for the day. We used to have these things, then they stopped. But we were listened to and we have these things back now. The artists have taken us to The Burrell Collection to let us have a look at the work there, and they took us to our art exhibitions in the airport and other museums and galleries in the city. If you don't get something, someone tells you why you didn't get it – like the art.

We're hoping to get a bigger art room, it's quite small. Once you've got four or five in there, it's quite tight. We were told we couldn't get bigger premises, so we accepted that. We did ask for a cabin in the yard, but that was put down because of the security and we'd need extra staff to staff it. We would need to convert maybe two rooms and that's a great expense right enough, but you can't think of that as money, because there's so much involved in it you know, in helping the patients. We realise it is probably a listed building and they wouldn't be allowed to do what they want, but it would be absolutely tremendous if we could get the funding, even to put another bit on the building somewhere to help us out.

It's a kind of partnership with the artists. We're always asked how we feel about this and that – they always ask you before they do anything. We're invited to bring in our own

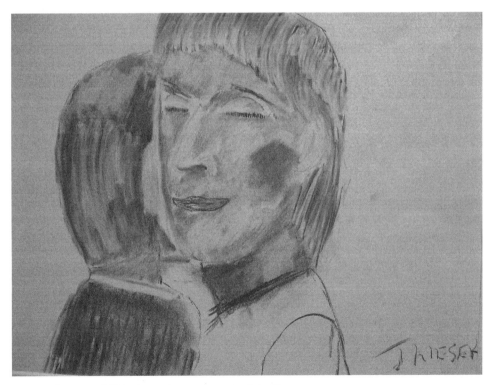

FIGURE 7 Dreamer, 2004, charcoal on canvas, by John Lieser.

music. We have exhibitions of our work and one day they came in and said that there would be an exhibition at Glasgow Airport and would we care to help select the paintings to be hung. I had done a portrait of my own wife and that was hanging in the exhibition. I was really proud of it. After the exhibition Marielle hung it in the snoozelum where we go for reflexology. The patients really liked it because they got a soothing feeling from the portrait. That's the type of things that happen here.

I'm still getting the benefit of the art. I'm still reaping the rewards of the effort I put in and I'm really hoping that it'll continue. My involvement in the development of hospice services, including the art and education, have really brought me out of myself. I wouldn't have survived without the hospice. Apart from my wife, they've done a lot of great things for me in here. It gives you a lot of hope and belief in yourself. If someone had said at the very beginning that you would have gone on and stood in front of a bunch of nurses and talked about this experience I couldn't have done that. Now I'd go all the way. I'd go anywhere just to get the point put over that we need art. If people were to come to me

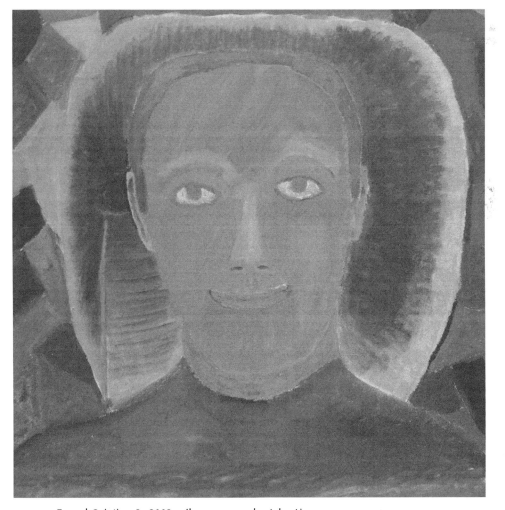

FIGURE 8 Tunnel Painting 2, 2002, oil on canvas, by John Lieser.

now and say 'John, would you do this' and 'John, would you do that', I would try it, I would definitely try it. It wouldn't matter what.

I don't want to keep the limelight, I'm not that kind of person. If patients were allowed to form a small committee of maybe three or four, even different people on different days, I think it would give the patients more confidence to give their ideas. I think we'd feel more involved as we'd not be sitting there getting told what to do. 'This is best for you.' The patients are asking in their own way what's best for them. That's more likely to happen because of the art. I know a number of people who would love to be on a committee. Maybe take one person out of each day and make a group up. You would get a different sort of look at the place, if everybody with different ideas came in and let the hospice know how they feel. I wouldn't like anybody to tell anyone what to do, it's not in my nature. Suggest, aye, suggest. That way I find that you still keep friendly with the people and people respect you a lot more, rather than saying, 'we want this' and 'we want that'. We don't want, we just suggest.

We would always need a member of staff to sit in with us in case a patient takes ill or something like that. But not to run the group – to advise us. The likes of how to go about it, how to get the right words to suit the occasion. Not everybody is clued up to that, they may say the wrong word and mean a different thing, so you'd be as well with a member of staff or even a volunteer to advise 'word it this way'. It's probably the best way it can be run, if the patients are involved they feel better within themselves.

I did a self portrait on what I thought about life when I was ill. It was a tunnel with a wee light at the end of the tunnel and that was how my life looked when I was ill. There was brick on the outside of the tunnel and everyone who helped me in the hospice, I put their initial on each brick, the doctors, the nurses, the volunteers, every one who had helped me through my illness. That's the way I seen my life, they were the foundation, as it were, for this tunnel with a wee light. A year later I did a painting, only this time I had come through the tunnel. It was a bright, bright tunnel with a wee, wee dark dot at the end of the tunnel. The same sort of painting but it was 'then' and 'now', as it were, and that's the best way I can describe what the art has done for my life. I've still got these paintings, they're up in Blawarthill Hospital and I always give them a wee look now and again to make me realise and pinch myself. I'm still here.

The hospice story

Arts in Palliative Care evolved from discussions between the Director of Cultural and Leisure Services at Glasgow City Council, the Scottish Arts Council and Art in Hospital – three organisations keen to redress an absence of quality, sustained arts provision within palliative care in Glasgow. In line with their priorities at the time, the Council funded the pilot for a comprehensive programme that would combine their objectives of enriching the quality of life and contributing to the improved health of the citizens of Glasgow, promoting social inclusion and equality of access to the arts and culture, and providing opportunities for lifelong learning. The findings supported a successful application to the Scottish Arts Council Lottery Fund. This process, including the time allocated for setting up the project and recruitment of the artist resulted in an eighteen-month gap in the workshop programme.

I met John halfway through his journey, during recruitment for the two-year Arts in Palliative Care project. Having worked extensively with individuals with challenging special educational needs, I was familiar with the potential of art to overcome physical limitations and communication issues and believed this would transfer to a palliative care setting. As an interviewee for my post, I had not shared John's bleak preconceptions of the hospice environment but had not anticipated the vibrant atmosphere and inherent community spirit of the Day Unit. The interview took place during a workshop to the accompaniment of a piano, violin and singing, all of which appeared to be initiated by patients. Despite the various distractions, John and a fellow participant sat studiously at the art table, testifying their conviction to the project and their rigorous campaign for its return. It was evident that art had made a profound impact on their lives, and with it, came an overwhelming sense of gratitude and relief.

During the pilot project the hospice was undergoing an extensive refurbishment programme. The in-patient unit and day services had subsequently been decanted to a local hospital ward and the pilot operated from a single table in a large communal room. This was instrumental in integrating the artists and in encouraging participation. When demand for the project exceeded expectations, it moved to an adjacent empty ward. This afforded a more appropriate workshop environment and a supportive group dynamic developed. Plans for the new purpose-built day unit had predated the pilot project and the traditional Georgian architecture of other areas presented access issues and growing demands from other care services. Arts in Palliative Care began as the pilot had done, at a single table in a corner of the day unit. Again, the social setting helped to build a regular clientele, with those who had attended the pilot continually canvassing for other participants. Whilst participation was encouraged through patients' own observations and our gentle persuasions as to the benefits and accessibility of arts activities, the role of other service users was paramount.

The location was still not conducive to a workshop programme of optimum therapeutic benefit to patients and I was concerned that the project would not progress from basic recreational activity. Restrictions on materials meant that those with poor motor skills or limited concentration and energy, could not benefit from messier, more immediate activities. Similarly, the power of artistic self-expression to bring meaning and empowerment to those with communication issues, could never truly be realised in such a socially vibrant and diverse environment. Instead, screened by an easel, art could be an alternative to communicating, rather than a vehicle for it. Moreover, a lack of privacy left people feeling exposed when creative activity had prompted significant emotional responses. The hospice presented an innovative solution in response to continuous requests from patients who had experienced the benefits of a dedicated art room during the pilot project. A substantial donation was allocated for the conversion of a bathroom on the ground floor and the art room was officially opened eight months into the project.

The move was met with some trepidation by patients and staff who had become accustomed to the project's presence as an activity for others to observe. Echoing the experiences of the pilot, these individuals felt deserted during workshops, owing to the growing popularity of the art project. Although the pilot had evidenced that appropriate accommodation was integral to therapeutic gain, some remained sceptical, perhaps as a result of the gap preceding the two-year project. However, the new art room realised the project's potential and subsequent patient feedback ensured all staff, clinical and non-clinical, recognised the arts project as intrinsic to patient care, as opposed to a luxury extension to hospice facilities or purely anecdotal. The invested enthusiasm strengthened ongoing attempts to secure essential funding where original match funding had fallen through. In addition, separate accommodation encouraged a wider audience, fulfilling the hospice's aim to provide valuable support for carers. Growing demand for the project has, as John implies, highlighted the need for larger premises. Responding to participants' needs, the hospice has identified alternative premises and is committed to the long-term fundraising required for the significant structural implications of such a project.

Excursions to augment and complement creative activities are integral to Art in Hospital's approach and were a prerequisite of Glasgow City Council's support for the project. This addressed patient requests for their reintroduction and encouraged the more reticent to suggest specific outings. Excursions are now part of day services' general activity programme, adhering to a new policy and procedure developed during Arts in Palliative Care, and evaluated by patients for continuous improvement. An extensive exhibition programme was organised in consultation with participants and, as John alludes to with his portrait of his wife, made a significant contribution to staff and patient morale. Acknowledging this and the potential for display of patients' art to imbue a sense of ownership, the hospice has allocated a significant donation for the development of an exhibition area. This will provide a permanent platform for participants to select and display the results of a project they have shaped from the outset.

After retiring, John Lieser was diagnosed with cancer in 1999 and given a prognosis of weeks. On subsequent referral to the Prince and Princess of Wales Hospice, Glasgow, he discovered painting through a pilot art project. Defying initial prognosis, he played a pivotal role in campaigning for permanent arts provision, the recruitment of staff and the allocation of a dedicated art room. Despite ongoing post radiotherapy problems with his speech, he became involved in professional education having gained confidence through art.

Marielle Macleman studied drawing and painting at Duncan of Jordanstone College of Art and Design, Dundee. After graduating in 1998, she worked as a freelance artist, continuing her own practice and delivering workshops in a variety of settings, focusing on special educational needs. Since joining Glasgow-based arts organisation Art in Hospital in 2003, she has co-ordinated the arts project at the Prince and Princess of Wales Hospice which presents a new model of arts in palliative care in Scotland.

CHAPTER 5

Connecting I and you: working with the breath as a tool to enable people to find their stories in safety

Lucinda Jarrett and Miranda Tufnell

The maxim of EM Forster's *Howard's End* is 'Only connect'. Writing at the turn of the century he used writing to attack a society increasingly divided by class, wealth, and industry. Working in palliative care, I often think of E M Forster as I try to meet the people who use the hospices without compassion or pity, so that we meet as equals and engage in creative activities as collaborative partners.

Rosetta Life was set up in 1997 to enable the dying to find the stories that matter and find a shape and form to express them. We work in partnership with over eighteen hospices and hospitals in England where we deliver arts residencies that culminate in events that celebrate the lives of those we work with.

As a person who works in a hospice, I am not a teacher who hands over the skills of a writer/filmmaker to a pupil, nor am I an artist interpreting another person's life. My role is to engage on a journey and accompany people as they find the stories and images that matter to them to enable them to celebrate their lives. Equally, the people I meet in the hospices struggle to overcome pain, fear, loss and loneliness to reach out to find the stories that matter to them and work with me to tell the stories that matter to them and their families to leave a lasting legacy.

This raises several ethical issues – what boundaries are in place if meetings take place as equals? Who owns copyright of the work? How do you enable people to access stories that matter to them and what censorship – if any – is imposed over the stories that are told. Each person we work with owns copyright of their work and if they choose, they bequeath to Rosetta Life the right to exhibit the work on a public website. This chapter focuses on one aspect of our work with patients – how we enable people to find stories that they own and that they can access without editorial censorship.

The finding of the stories is the most important part of our work. We avoid stories that are the narrative of medical illness and the stories of memory and reminiscence, but seek to find the stories that celebrate the vitality of people's lives in the present. We seek the stories of our senses. This chapter is the story of the search for a process that will aid artists working in palliative care and the growth of a practice. This is the story of how two women connected to work together with movement and breath to enable the dying and those facing death to access their stories.

Lucinda Jarrett:
I met Jimmy in March 2002. He closed his eyes and we breathed together. I watched his breath and waited until I found his rhythm and took on his breathing pattern. I asked him to wait until he felt supported and then to open his eyes. A few minutes later he opened his eyes and began to speak of his love of photography and how working as a press photographer had destroyed his love of image and photograph. ' I want to find happiness again', he said. 'I want to find happiness by rediscovering my love of light.' The next week we met and I followed the rhythm of his breath again. Before he opened his eyes he began to speak about light and what it meant to him. The next week we went to Highgate Woods and photographed the light in the trees and as he took the photographs he described to me how he searched and found the frame for each image and why he was choosing certain images over others. Over the next few months, we compiled a set of photographs and with the help of the partner of a nurse at the hospice we were able to make sure that they were framed in English oak, and then exhibited them at the hospice that he attended. His photographs remained exhibited on the wall outside the doctor's office for many months after he died at the hospital.

All our stories are held in our body, not the physical body but the sensing body of our felt experiences. The supported rhythm of his breath enabled Jimmy to travel inside his body without the fear of looking at tumour and cancer. He was focused upon inhalation and exhalation. He found the story himself because I was not a mediator/interpreter but accompanied him through breath and movement to the place he chose to rest.

As an artist the focus is always on the making of the work. This means that the 'boundaries' in place are themselves the form and the shape of the work. Accessing the stories is an open process. This opening to the sensory world is unboundaried and uncensored.

'I was so scared. I was so scared of losing you. I thought you might not make it. I was so frightened and alone when you had the chemotherapy. I hated being apart.'

A young boy wrote this about his fear of losing his mother. Every day in the hospice movement I encounter people living with fear and am struck by the difficulty we face sitting alongside fear without needing to 'make it better'. I sit with people, find the rhythm of their breath and in supporting the rhythm of breath support the person.

In
Out
In
Out
In

Entrance and exit; inhalation and exhalation; the renewal and exhaustion of oxygen; the cycle of birth and death are all held in the process of breathing. The process of breath is the connection between the body and the environment. This connection can provide a profound support. Maybe the connection itself, the support of the breath between one person and another is a boundary that guides the practice. It provides the perimeter of our travelling.

The fear that the young boy spoke of is the fear of existential isolation. The loneliness of an orphaned child. Working with the breath enables us to counter fear of loneliness with connectivity between the self and the landscape and others within it. Opening ourselves to the landscape makes us feel participants in the landscape instead of isolated individuals. We connect with the sound of the wind, the birds, the stream of traffic and in so doing our bodies' senses are awakened to the stories that these experiences offer.

The phenomenologist, Edmund Husserl, provides us with evidence and support for this theory. He argued that we should understand perception not as subject and object, or 'I' and 'you' but as the experiential reality of a sensed world. Merlau Ponty took this theory further and argued for a participatory understanding of perception. He sought 'recognition for the sensing body, ceaselessly spreading out of itself as well as breathing in the world'.

Rosetta Life was set up as a partnership between a movement therapist, Filipa Pereira Stubbs, and myself – writer, producer and theatre maker. Since its inception, we have been exploring ways to access the active imagination, the organic and felt experience of our lived relationships. It was not until I met Miranda Tufnell that we were able to take the philosophy of phenomenology and connect this with movement and story in a radical form.

Miranda Tufnell:
I first met Lucinda Jarrett at a workshop I was leading in Oxford on body and imagination, a workshop using movement, writing and making to explore the landscapes of dreams. Lucinda and I talked together in the breaks, she described her own process of working in palliative care, her sense that movement sourced in the sensing, feeling body could enable a person facing the end of their life to find the language necessary to express their life story. That at the end of life how vital that the failing body was engaged in the search for expression and meaning. Lucinda's dedication profoundly touched me. Her concern that there should be work in and with the body at such a time overlapped my own working.

When I met Lucinda in the autumn of 2000 I had spent nearly 30 years exploring how to support the body to find its own voice – movement, the language of the body and a way of tracking the moment by moment flow of sensation and feeling. Movement sourced in this way seemed to connect body and soul and bring to the surface images and stories that held a sense of personal significance and value. I accompanied Lucinda several times to her group sessions at a hospice in Hampstead. Her capacity to bring awareness to the physical body through breath offered a profound and centring means for each person involved to connect to what really mattered for them.

Lucinda Jarrett:
In Spring 2003 I ran a very small movement group for people attending a hospice in North London for six weeks. We would breathe together and, working in pairs, find the support of a partner's breath and then move spontaneously from a sitting position, allowing the breath to lead the movement. Then we would take time to draw freely and explore in pairs the stories of the images. Images of laughter, solitude, trees, landscape of ferns and hills, rivers and mountains instigated stories of childhood re-experienced in the present, favourite places, metaphor, poetry and symbol. The natural world was the dominant source of all imagery. Connecting with place was significant even for those who had spent all their lives in an inner city environment.

One woman drew the sea again and again and then spoke about trying to use the rhythm of breath and the sea as a way of finding peace in meditation. Constantly concerned about her inability to reach God behind the business of a distracted and fearful mind, she wrote the following poem.

Reaching God Behind Enemy Lines

Daniel was a man of prayer
But I'm not regular about the time.
It's six o'clock and I'm muddled and feeling quite dense.
Where is He, for goodness sake?
Could he be very busy,
As my Catholic friend sometimes says?

Let me try to begin with the sound of the sea
The gentle lapping where first contact began,
Like the kindness of my mother's voice –
But she when provoked could turn angry too
Storms and chaos in nature
Appear to reflect the emotions of men,
Making it difficult sometimes
To make contact with God.

Why is there always warfare?
In peacetime it is easier to find our God.
Even Daniel's faith could not provide direct access
Many years ago a Persian Spirit or prince
Stopped an angel providing a swift response
To answer Daniel's prophetic dreams.

Perhaps I am in a muddle again
With thoughts that are difficult to speak.
I need a free mind to meditate.
It is a long path to clear before I reach God.

A young man used the rhythm of breath to find again the vitality of life. A few days before he died he came to a session and drew a series of arcs that reached higher and higher on the page as if he was drawing the strength of his spirit through his breath.

The clarity with which people articulated their stories gave me the confidence to commission a dance performance from Miranda Tufnell about the processes of awakening stories. We hoped that the dance performance would take some steps towards explaining this new practice. I hoped that the performance would enable the participants to find their own stories and images and to enable an audience to reach a common understanding of humanity perceived through the ordinariness of lived experience at the end of life.

This was the first time we had ever asked people to participate in a process that would acknowledge their stories but would be owned by the artists creating the piece. This was a very difficult transition. We arranged for Miranda Tufnell, musician Sylvia Hallett and filmmaker Simon Hyde to run six workshops that would provide the stories that would form the content of the piece. Miranda and Sylvia and Simon's role was to honour that content in a creative work that would celebrate their humanity and pay tribute to the processes that had awakened the stories.

Miranda Tufnell:

After several times of meeting and working together Lucinda asked me and a close friend and musician colleague, Sylvia Hallett to work with people at St Thomas's day hospice and to make a performance that would in some way celebrate the lives of those involved in the project. And so for six Thursday mornings Sylvia and I, together with a video artist from Rosetta Life, Simon Hyde, visited the Dimbleby Day Centre. Over those few weeks we gathered material from writings, conversations, drawings and movement, slowly stories, memories, observations and laughter emerged and were shared. And something personal from each person's words and 'story 'was recorded. In response we took in stones, feathers, pictures of galaxies, of birds, of trees, to give tangible form to some of the images and dreams expressed by participants.

The group varied from week to week as members' health fluctuated. The centre itself was to close in the following month and the group dispersed so there was doubled poignancy to the meetings. Despite this the generosity and tenderness of each member of the group towards each other, and towards us as outsider artists was humbling. They must have wondered what we would do with their words, their stories, and we felt touched by the trust and openness with which people engaged with our sessions.

Each meeting began with a gathering together in a seated circle, greetings all around and then quiet, eyes closed and a relaxation and visualisation following some aspect of breath in the body. This was following work already initiated by Lucinda. Gradually we invited letting the hands imagine the feel of breath and to express that movement. It was beautiful to watch peoples faces soften as they became absorbed, hands rose and fell, opened, hovered, reached or closed inwards.

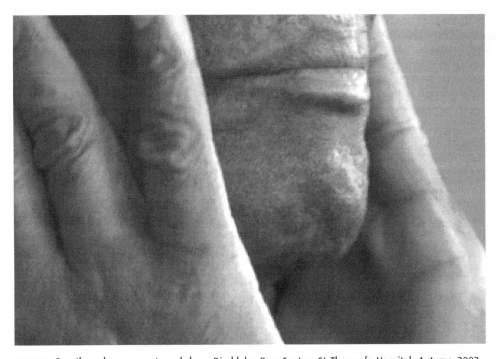

FIGURE 9 Breath and movement workshop, Dimbleby Day Centre, St Thomas's Hospital, Autumn 2003.

Sylvia's sound both followed and inspired, offering different textures and qualities. In the wake of moving we would each write, draw or simply talk in small groups to share the images and reveries that had surfaced. The wordlessness of movement awakens and reveals forgotten parts of ourselves that in turn changes and enlivens the familiar stories we tell about ourselves. It is often difficult to know what we feel, to sift and name the differing strands that compose our feelings, hard to find a language adequate for our experience, to say really what we mean.

Yet as human beings we need to communicate who and how we are, and to communicate dimensions of ourselves that are often inaccessible to language. Moving in the rhythm of the breath quietens the mind, and allows mind and body to hear each other and to connect more fully to what is around us.

In December and January Sylvia, Simon and myself worked in Cumbria to begin a shaping of material. How could we convey the wonderful sense of living, not of dying, we had found at the day hospice, the way the people treasured the ordinary details of their lives, meetings with friends, holidays by the sea, from the mundane getting up, washing, shaving, to the delight of sunlight warming the face and a sense of mystery and transcendence.

Projecting the image of an absent person is a curious and problematic experience. How could we avoid a sense of exposure, betrayal of intimacy, for those whose words and bodies we had recorded, even though permission had been given at every point? Over the days of working together we immersed ourselves in the voices and images of this group of people and found ourselves increasingly touched and moved by the sense of intimacy, familiarity. We came to know and love each person's voice, face and gesture, yet they did not see or hear of us, had no control over what we might do with their words. As we watched the video or listened to taped conversations we realised how complex and challenging this process of recording, editing was going to be.

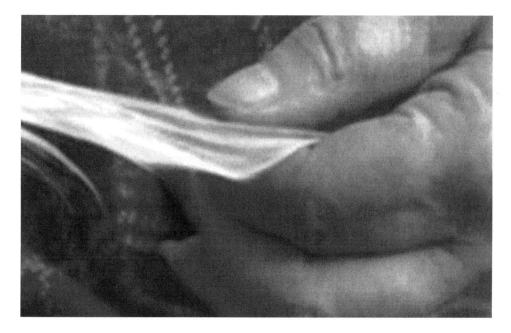

FIGURE 10 Playing with feathers in breath and movement workshop, Dimbleby Day Centre, St Thomas's Hospital, Autumn 2003.

Gradually we built up a bank of visual images to mix with footage of the group talking, laughing or moving – images that we hoped would evoke the landscapes of memory and feeling people had shared with us – a flying cormorant, winter trees, leaves in sunlight, waves on a shore line, people walking in streets, swans on a river. Every image inevitably invoked a cascade of other associations whose impact we needed to be aware of. In January we returned with the beginnings of a piece which all the group saw and felt able to comment on. That way we shared ownership, gave something back by way of celebrating their lives. Their responses to the work were recorded on audio and these were used in the final soundscape that Sylvia created to accompany the video sequences of images and the movement of the dancer. We spent the next three months working together to create the final performance. We were constantly aware of the other people in the rehearsal room, constantly aware that our role was not to interpret their humanity but to offer it as a gift to the audience. Breath was performed at Riverside Studios, July 2004. All those who had participated in the workshops came to the final performance in July. Their voices and faces dominated the stage projections and people were pleased to recognise their contributions to the piece.

Lucinda Jarrett:
We learnt many lessons from the performance of Breath in a public arts venue. We learnt to work with people in palliative care and enable them to find support from the sensory landscape they found themselves in. We learnt to feel connected. Held by the breath as if it were substantial matter.

Most significant were the simple lessons. The ethics of access in theatre are difficult to negotiate. The theatre has wheelchair access but not all hospice users chose to come in wheelchairs and none brought cushions with them. This may sound inconsiderable but it meant that their experience of the theatre was tarnished by discomfort. Our learning was that in order to honour those participants we must make sure that venues are not only accessible but comfortable. We must also offer public arts and performance tours to hospices where transport, access and comfort are more easily provided.

The next performance we worked on was at St Thomas's Hospital in partnership with a breast cancer support group for newly diagnosed women. Support is offered to women who are often receiving treatment for primary breast cancer which has the potential to be curable. There are 41 000 women diagnosed with breast cancer per year (latest figs) and 13 000 die of breast cancer per year. There are a lot of women living with breast cancer. Even without treatment, women with breast cancer are likely to live on average five years, and with treatment most women live over 15 years as it is a slowly developing disease and many people don't die of it, but go on to die of other causes – and the median age to get it is 64.

It is therefore unsurprising that this group is one of the longest running support groups in the country. Support groups offer people a safe place to talk and can also forge a collective voice or create a strong sense of affirmation for those involved. It was the latter that led me to propose a creative project that would offer to those interested a public platform for their voice. I also hoped that some women would be well enough to participate in a final performance that they could more fully and completely own. In March 2005 I began working with a group of women living with breast cancer.

I made a decision to programme the work in an intimate studio space that would not be intimidating for those participating, where the venue was a local venue for all women and therefore easy to access for friends and family, and we made it clear that people could bring cushions to make themselves comfortable. We were thrilled when Southwark Playhouse accepted the performance for their Spring programme.

Workshops began with simple walking through the space. We used the same space where the support group was held but opened out the space to make it wider. People identified one end of the room for their 'therapy' or 'support group' and the other end for the room for their 'creative support'. We found lots of ways to connect with each other and with our wider society: on one occasion we found a space next to the window that overlooked the river and used a visualisation to connect us to the river and the landscape of the open sea. On other occasions we talked about families, loss, longing and drew and wrote about our experiences.

We explored the floor, worked with visualisation and breath as tools to access image. Over the course of the next few weeks we became braver with the use of movement. Working in partners we walked with eyes closed, walked in pairs with one person's eyes closed and the other acting as guide through the touch of fingertips.

From the outset it was clear that people wanted to make a public performance that would articulate how people had experienced the threat of death while living with breast cancer. Image was very important, images of isolation, loneliness and hope were always articulated through placing people in landscapes that were real and imagined. One woman was very frightened of her cancer and was undergoing surgery for a double mastectomy while we were working together. She saw her role as supporting the other women arriving at a safe place to build a new life. After dancing she drew an image of an open landscape with a broad sky. 'I cannot believe I am here' she wrote in the corner, 'this familiar landscape with my feet on the ground and the wind above the sand dunes.' Here with her feet on the ground – a place she never expected to be, dancing reconnected her with her living experiencing body and made her feel alive.

Later we handed out disposable cameras to all the women to find photographic images in the landscape for the images they had found while dancing. The same woman went to the park and took a photo of the deer. She took a photo of the deer very close to her. Later she explained, 'they made me feel less alone. As though the world was bigger than me. I found that reassuring. I was in their world but part of it and not alone in it'. The following week she brought in this song:

I feel the warmth of the sun on my face
As I walk in the deer park, my special place

Here the deer roam freely without a care
So can I – they barely notice I'm there

Breathing the beauty of the deer and the trees
There's more out there in the world than me

So let's make the most of every day
Let's cherish the laughs we have on the way

The song was set to music and performed in the production that opened at Southwark Playhouse, 5–8 April 2006. We rehearsed for two weeks with musician Tea Hodzic and choreographers and dance makers Lucia Walker and Miranda Tufnell. It was wonderful to watch the performers become more confident both on stage and embodied in their language and their movement.

It was important to recognise that performance is not for everyone and that as people make the journey back to work rehearsals and performances become difficult to fit into a working schedule. Many of the women who participated in the workshops performed live on stage. Some chose to participate through digital voice recordings.

Conclusion

When it comes to an awareness of the sensory and imaginative presence of our own bodies, many of us draw a peculiar blank – as if we were anaesthetised from that which is closest and most vital to us. This lack of awareness within our own bodies limits our entire sense of ourselves, as sentient and feeling beings.

Imagery, story, and metaphor which are the heart of arts practice all invoke the senses. Creative work in the arts (and in a broader sense our creative way of being in the world) is to an important degree sourced in the sensory awareness of the body. All the arts draw upon the senses and the senses themselves are rooted in the body. We must learn to find ways to embrace and celebrate the stories our bodies hold both in movement and in stillness. Through this more personal and 'embodied' approach to the imagination we learn to forge our own meaning in things and this in turn affects our health and sense of connectedness to the world around us.

This work is of particular validity within the hospice movement where palliative care is practised holistically and where care of the social, psychological, spiritual and physical well being is rooted in multidisciplinary practice. Visualisation, image work and meditation and relaxation are already embraced as principles of palliative care and working more imaginatively with the body is a small step for many practitioners to embrace.

For artists working in healthcare, working with dance offers a way to connect and imagine in a place of safety and trust. The relationship between artist and person who uses the hospice service/hospital service is one that is fragile. Many medical models find this difficult and challenging to embrace. However, by working with breath and movement there is a connected channel that enables service users to trust the relationship itself as a source of support and a place of safety. This openness to the sensory world becomes a supportive one.

It is clear that this creative practice needs further research if it is to be disseminated. However, embracing dance and movement in palliative care could prove to be critical to developing user involvement principles. It enables us to develop a symbolical language of personal imagery and could help us to develop a language for death and dying that is creative and challenges the contemporary words that prevail. The Living Body Project is a loose alliance formed by Miranda Tufnell between performance practitioners, writers, psychotherapists and artists working in healthcare and scientists who are committed to develop understanding of the living body through direct participation with sensation, feeling, movement and image in order to raise awareness and open up new areas of research and practice in health, education and the arts.

Miranda Tufnell has been working as a dancer and choreographer since 1976. She trained in Alexander Technique and craniosacral therapy in order to develop a deeper understanding of what is sensed and known in the body. She has worked part time in the NHS for fourteen years and has co-authored two books with Chris Crickmay, *Body, Space and Image* and *A Widening Field: Journeys in Body and Imagination.*

Lucinda Jarrett is artistic director of Rosetta Life, an artist-led organisation that delivers artist-led residencies in hospices and hospitals across England. She founded the organisation in 1997 in order to challenge our contemporary representation of illness and to enable people who are facing death to participate more fully in cultural life.

Lucinda read English and theatre at Edinburgh University and then studied the semiotics of dance at the University of Paris. She worked in television for five years where she worked as assistant television producer for French, American and British broadcasters, and has written and performed performance poetry across London venues. She is a published writer and has worked with independent dance venues and independent dancers and has a strong track record of delivering theatre within healthcare settings.

CHAPTER 6

We laughed

A collaboration between Billy Bragg and Maxine Edgington

In October 2005 Rosetta Life released three songs on a CD. Billy Bragg wrote the following introduction to the songs:

The songs were the product of a series of song-writing workshops I conducted at the Trimar Hospice in Weymouth during February 2005. I was invited to take part in the project by Rosetta Life, a charity dedicated to helping those facing terminal illness to share their experiences through the medium of art, poetry, film or song. My work was part of a larger project called Rosetta Requiem, commissioned by Culture Online, which aims to challenge the way in which we think about death.

Every Friday morning for six weeks, I worked with half a dozen women who came to the hospice for palliative care as they fought against the effects of breast cancer. Maxine Edgington had the clearest idea of what she wanted to do. In our first one-on-one session, she pulled a picture out of her bag and said 'Look, I've been given six months to live. I don't want to mess about. I want to write the song of this picture.'

When her condition was diagnosed in November 2004, Maxine's thoughts turned immediately to how she would be remembered, particularly by her fifteen-year-old daughter, Jessica. Determined that Jess should have positive memories of her after the grieving

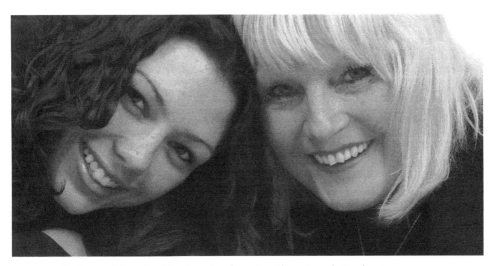

FIGURE 11 Maxine and her daughter Jess laughing together at a photo shoot.

was over, Maxine commissioned a professional photo shoot which produced beautiful images of mother and daughter smiling together, looking as thought they had not a care in the world. This was how she wanted to be remembered. As Maxine says 'Cancer is terrible, but at least it gives you the chance to put things right with those you love.'

Maxine wrote reams of words, pouring her feelings out onto the page. My job was to take the words that best expressed the sentiments in the photographs and shape them into a song. I provided the melody, but the words were Maxine's. She called the song 'We Laughed'.

In June, I got together with some local musicians and we recorded this CD. The additional tracks feature lyrics written by Lisa Payne and Veronica Barfoot, who also took part in the workshops. That there is not a shred of pity or morbidity in any of these songs is a testament to the spirit of these three women. I found the experience of collaborating with them to be inspirational.

You can go to www.rosettarequiem.org to find out more about how Maxine and I wrote the song. The site also features short film clips of us talking about the process.

Money raised by the sale of the song will go to Rosetta Life, the Trimar Hospice and the hospice users who contributed to this CD.

God's glory revealed

Maxine Edgington

The diary of a process
On 30 November 2004 I was told that I was terminally ill with cancer and had six months or less to live.

I had had cancer in August 2000. I had had both breasts removed. This second breast cancer was not from the original cancer. This cancer was actually a different type of breast cancer. It was a very aggressive cancer. The cancer had initially grown in the chest wall, but had already spread as secondary carcinomas into the lung in six places and into the lymph system. It was so extensive that it was not curable. I was offered palliative care.

Great! I thought, How could someone with both breasts removed get another type of breast cancer! So what were my options now? Well, the one option that seemed clear was that the next stage was going to take me to meet Jesus in Heaven.

Not that I did not want to see my Lord and Saviour. I actually had no problem with that. Only I did not want to die. I have a daughter of fifteen and I did not want to leave her. I did not want to have any of her future stolen either. For her to be left without her mother would have been a huge loss for her. Why should I be removed off this earth before I have finished my life and what I needed to do in it? I am a single parent and just felt so backed into a corner that I was trapped. I felt very vulnerable and out of control.

I have no fear of death and had not had for many years. I had made many decisions in 2000, when I had faced cancer before, that helped me now in my fight against this second cancer. However, this situation was totally different. Either God was going to heal me or I would die. I had no secondary plan. My body was already racked in pain and deteriorating physically through the cancer.

I was determined to have the number of days that were allocated to me. I was not going to be short changed. I was going to have all the time that I believed was mine and for my daughter Jessica.

I had no problem in believing in a miracle. I wanted the miracle from the moment I found out I was terminal. That was spiritually what I wanted, yet I knew it was God's decision. It was his choice. It was all down to him.

I was out of control and God was in control. That was a strange feeling. This time God was asking for the most precious area of my life. My daughter and her future without me. On the outside it all appeared so bleak. Yet I had an overwhelming feeling that every thing was going to be all right.

Moreover, there was something in me that mentally could not believe any of what my specialist oncologist was saying. I had all sorts of people from cancer care and social services helping me. I went into Joseph Weld Hospice, Dorset to get the morphine and numerous other drugs stabilised and I began to meet the staff who would be responsible for my palliative care until I died. I had a few days to deal with the physical shock. I also started to visit the Trimar Hospice in Weymouth once a week for my pain control and special care. I had been to the day hospice in 2000 and knew what they offered. I was pleased to go and to utilise the service. The same nurse who helped me in 2000 was now helping me again. Wendy knew me very well and never questioned my belief that I wanted the miracle. She always said that if any one can fight this with their belief and faith in God, it was me. She gave me hope.

People were openly talking about what my needs would be for the short period of time that I had to live. As they were sorting out a specialised chair, bed and other things that I required physically, I had a sense of unreality. Mentally I kept thinking that all these professionals were talking about someone else. I guess it could have been said that I was in denial.

I look back and realise that my mind was unable to accept reality. I remember thinking, 'Once these professionals find out I am not dying, then I am going to be in so much trouble. I will end up in prison. They are giving me all this physical and financial support and there is nothing wrong with me'. I actually felt like a fraud. However, I needed a full-time carer, as my strength was departing rapidly. I was losing weight very quickly. I needed the specialised things they were providing as I could no longer get on and off the settee and in and out of the bath. I was unable to get out of bed without the lift.

I was in major turmoil. I was on a rollercoaster ride. A white-knuckle ride that I had not even asked for.

I felt that six months was not very much time to put right what had taken me 47 years to get wrong. I also felt that six months was not enough time to change any thing that needed to be changed. What difference could I make in six months. I had an overwhelming desire to get things in order. Mentally and spiritually. I do not believe that any one can face death and not think about meeting God and putting their life in order. God told me that he was concerned about my cancer. He was only concerned with making me a whole person.

I have to say that I found this very confusing at first. I remember thinking,

'Well, you may not be concerned about the cancer but I am!'

I went to the Trimar Hospice where I also met Catherine and we discussed the opportunity of working with Billy Bragg. I was very sceptical as I thought that I had other things to do that needed major attention. Such as finding someone who would look after my daughter and be her guardian after I had gone.

However I was drawn to the project and I am so pleased that the opportunity arose, and that I was one of the people chosen to take part because it was the opening of the doorway that I needed.

God works in mysterious ways and Billy Bragg was in His plan for me. The song writing project gave me the creative opportunity that was going to be a doorway to freedom and hope for me. Using the writing of the song as a tool or vehicle I was able to think and write about all aspects of my life. I was able to be honest. I was able to be free. Creativity has no boundaries and no rules. So I did not have to be any thing else except me. Strange how strange that is. Even now I expect it has some technical name – poetic licence or something. It felt astonishing to be able to write intimate things about myself without imposing any restrictions. It gave me the feeling that I had no fear and nothing to lose.

These were big steps that I was taking. I was walking towards the whole person that God had asked me to become.

In my creative writing I was able to own some of the situations that I had been responsible for that had been part of my 'colourful' life. I understood the hurt that they had caused me and became whole through owning them and then facing the reality of what I had done.

In the writing of the song I was able to get a balance. I was able to see that it was not all bad and that so many things I had done had been right and so many things that I had done with Jessica I would want to do again. I saw that there were some wonderful things that had developed out of the chaotic lifestyle that I had led. That there was an enormous amount of laughter. I was pleased to find the balance.

I also found myself in a position of having nothing else to prove. I had always thought that I had to prove my Christianity and what a good Christian I was. I always thought that I had to prove I was a good parent, a good mother, a good person. Although I appeared to be confident, I always had low self-esteem. Song writing set me free. I just had nothing to prove in my life. I felt whole.

I felt very different and in a position of strength. Silly really, when I was terminal. Mentally something happened that I cannot explain. I was just in another dimension of faith, of belief, and there was no looking back.

I did accept that I had to give her to God and, as much as I wanted to stay with her to be a part of her future, I accepted that if I died I would have no influence over Jess at all. I had to trust God with her future and her life. Eventually, after three days of arguing with God, I finally gave my Daughter to Him. I came to understand that no other human being could love her more than me and that emotion was written into the song. My heart strings broke. The pain was terrible. It was a physical pain. It was probably the lowest point of my illness.

I handed Jessica over to the Father's hands.

I gave Him my all.

I had nothing more precious than her in my life.

I lay in bed in the middle of the night in the darkness and I imagined God with his huge hand outstretched. The hands that flung stars into space and made the world. The all powerful God. Yet the gentle God who loves and cares for Jess and I. I put her into His hands and knew that I had to leave her with Him. Who else could I trust her with?

The next morning I then felt complete freedom. I felt relief. I felt that my daughter was safe regardless of me. For the first time in my life I could be me. I wrote the last part of the song. I put you in the Father's hands.

I was mentally blessed. Somehow in the freedom of the creativity of writing this song with Billy Bragg I had found the freedom to become whole. A whole person.

I found the strength then to fight the cancer.

I refused to allow any thoughts of self-pity. I refused to go into thoughts of depression or dark thoughts of what was going to happen to Jess if I did die.

I knew my mind must focus on those things that are good and wholesome. That I had many things to think about that were good. They were all in the song.

I had seen and have been familiar with cancer all my life. I have a genetic cancer that has been passed down from generation to generation and my great grandmothers and grandmothers, mother, aunts and sisters have died from it. I grew up with all the women in my family dying from cancer. I had the privilege of nursing my sister, Christine, through her illness. She died 11 years ago at the age of 43. Cancer is an illness I know well.

Cancer is also an illness that Jess knows well. As our lives move on, we face an uncertain future. We do not know whether Jess has the gene or not. I do not know who is going to teach Jess better than me how to fight this horrible disease. I thank God that he has allowed me to stay around to do that. Cancer is an illness that holds no fear for me now. I have faced it, fought it and moved on.

Every day that I am alive over the six months that I was given is a miracle. I see that as the truth and a fact. That is how I think. I think that I have had a miracle. The inevitable has been put off and today and every day that I wake up and am alive is a holiday. Yes it feels like a big holiday.

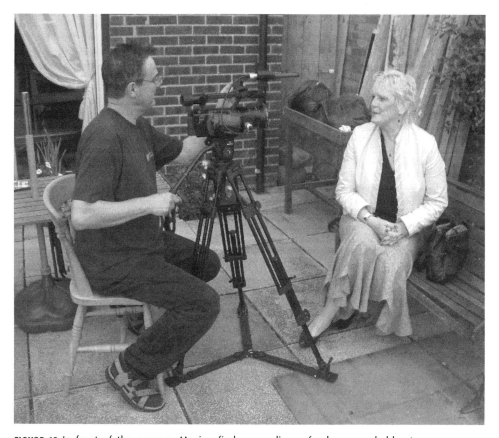

FIGURE 12 In front of the camera. Maxine finds an audience for her remarkable story.

I love the song that has been written and I love the words and music. Billy Bragg is a very special person in my life and I have no idea how to thank him. Rosetta Life offers people who have life-threatening illnesses a unique opportunity. It has been a very special experience for me.

The hospice story

The following entries are taken from Catherine Batten's diary of the process of working with Billy Bragg at Trimar Hospice, Weymouth.

Friday 4 February 2005

Billy Bragg at Trimar went well. In the afternoon, talked to Maxine. She had been given six months to live three months ago and is having chemo for what was a huge lump that has now reduced. The chemo is making her very sick. In 2000 she had a double mastectomy and reconstruction using her stomach muscles. She has a 15-year-old daughter, Jessica. She is a devout Christian and is 'praying for a miracle'. I suggested the possibility of her making a video diary with her daughter. Afterwards I felt quite upset and difficult about what she had told me, I think because of our similar ages, only daughters and being single parents ... too much to identify with.

Monday 7 February 2005

A report from staff of some resistance to the Billy Bragg session from patients on the way home on the bus, but am not too worried as the direct feedback was positive and it is very early days ...

Friday 11 February 2005

Towards the end, Maxine and Lisa went into the art room to have individual sessions with Billy. I didn't follow with the camera as I felt it would be intrusive at this early stage, and that the women should have time and space to gain confidence in Billy and themselves in the song writing process. However, from the feedback, both from Billy and the girls, it sounds as if it went very well and I feel very impressed by and envious of the way Billy was able to work with them both.

Friday 25 February 2005

Max only came in briefly as she is feeling very sick with the chemo, but she has brought in several pages of thoughts and feelings for Billy to work from. She is really struggling with what the writing is bringing up for her – she was tearful and emotional and said that she didn't feel up to doing a session with Billy ... despite this she did spend some time with him ...

Friday 4 March 2005

Billy came in and worked with everyone again ... spoke to him afterwards, he says that he's totally inspired by working with the women. It takes him days to come back to earth after each session and he is getting a huge amount from them ... he seemed to really want to talk about it ...

Billy Bragg was described by *The Times* as a 'national treasure'. In the two and a half decades of his career Bragg has certainly made an indelible mark on the conscience of British music, becoming perhaps the most stalwart guardian of the radical dissenting tradition that stretches back over centuries of the country's political, cultural and social history.

Maxine Edgington was a service user at Trimar Hospice, Weymouth. She died in March 2006.

Catherine Batten is Rosetta Life artist in residence at Trimar Hospice, Weymouth. She also works with West Dorset Food and Land Trust where she co-ordinates the Bridport Local Food Heritage Project.

PART 2: **DEVELOPING SUPPORT**

Meet my cancer Mel Anoma
You can call him Mel.
He's very close to me.
We're inseparable, in fact.
Ever the enthusiast, trying to get out.
And about seven years
I've kept him hidden.
Mrs. Rochester, in my liver, waiting for the moment,
His time in the winter sun.
Mel's real feisty. Won't-take-no-for-an-answer.
Just because I want to be your friend, I say, doesn't mean I have to like what you're
   doing.
Eating my liver, school dinner crunchy.
Will turn me yellow in time.
Doesn't he know that's Norwich City?
Maybe if I'm nice he'll make it Ipswich-Town-Away-Strip orange.
He's not really shy.
He's hidden depths.
You have to speak quietly, that's all.
Ranting just makes him mad (not good for a psychiatrist.)
Mel Liffluous is the voice.
Seductive. Makes me <u>hot</u>.
The bed clothes I've soaked...but just with sweat.
[Kids go 'Eeeuw'
We all go 'Eeeuw']
He's a quieter laugh.
Low Butthead giggle.
'Look what I make you do'
Mel makes me:
Live* with exhilaration
Live** with exhilaration
Insane with senses
The best porridge in the world.
Vietnam Ted has lived on the edge of death
But only half an hour at a time.
Suicide bombers are as blessed as me: a serene flash of expiration.

Ultraviolet ultra-violence.
Could you use me Mel Anoma, the MI6 mole?

Meet my cancer, Mel Anoma.
Thinks he's smart to make me Homer.
Screaming yellows from wife and kids.
The bastard hostage taker!
I <u>will</u> negotiate. No terror.
Calm. Calm. Have water. Have food.
Die of obesity.
Mel's my friend.
What happens to him, goes for me too.
Till I'm gone.

Paul Laking
December 2004

60

CHAPTER 7

User involvement and creativity

Nuala Cullen and David Alcock

This chapter is divided into two sections. The first looks at the relationship between user involvement and creativity in theory and in practice. The second describes a creative project and illustrates the power and influence that people have over the creative work that they do.

Part 1: the relationship between user involvement and creativity

Nuala Cullen

I was asked to contribute to this chapter at a very timely moment for the hospice in which I am a social worker. Creativity and user involvement, in the form of user groups, are being embraced as separate issues which aim to bring further value to the experience of the people who come to the hospice and use our services. When I was asked to write a chapter, which suggests a marriage between these two areas, several assumptions were revealed in my mind and have challenged me in my thoughts and forward planning for user involvement.

My assumptions can be briefly condensed as follows: creativity is exciting, energetic and imaginative. User involvement is dry, onerous and limited in its impact. I have been energetic in my desire to see a creative project evolve at the hospice where I work, but have procrastinated and delayed 'grasping the nettle' of user groups. How, I thought, is it possible for these two areas to meet and have a beneficial relationship with each other? I will start by outlining my view about the context of palliative care from my position as a social worker. I will address my ideas about the value of creativity and then explore ways in which it might lend itself to, and enhance the value of, user involvement. I will then look at the concepts of 'Voice' and 'Identity', which may be revealed to be the key common factors to impact on the relationship between creativity and user involvement. By embracing creativity, we encourage and value the voice of the person. We encourage people to express externally what is internal in their thoughts, feelings, being and self. This acknowledgement of the person, behind the 'patient' label, changes the nature of the person's relationship with an organisation, particularly in the context of health organisations and the experience of having a 'patient' label. Ultimately, this maximises the opportunity for the person to be empowered so that they could contribute their voice to hospice ownership and development.

Palliative care: the context

Palliative care embraces holistic care as a defining idea. This means that a person may meet the service as a result of a relationship with life-limiting illness, but this person need not be identified as a primarily 'medical being'. Indeed, this person may not necessarily be the person with the illness in their body. Holistic care acknowledges that the illness 'happens' not only to the 'patient', but impacts on their network of family and friends, and looks to recognise their individual needs in a meaningful way. As a human being, the 'person' can also be a social being, an emotional being, a creative being, a spiritual being, a financial being, and so on. This is determined by our changing relationships with our 'self', our network of family and friends, and the illness that has brought palliative care into life.

The value of creativity

If palliative care is understood within the context that I have outlined above, what value does creativity have in contributing to the holistic nature of this care? The unique position of creativity that stands apart from other elements of holistic care is that it works solely, and collaboratively, from an agenda that is determined by the person. Creative expression can be defined as a story-telling experience, with the story being chosen by the teller. It can be the process of unravelling a story rather than the end result that holds the most therapeutic value. Ownership of creative expression, or story, belongs to the storyteller, as do decisions about sharing the story.

The aim of user involvement

User involvement seeks to acknowledge ownership by people who use services and to encourage their input into dialogue about their experiences with those services and about organisational development. This is a particularly pertinent exercise when looking at services of organisations in the voluntary sector, especially when these organisations are localised in the way that hospices are. In a very real way, one can clearly see how local communities contribute, through their charitable input, to the hospices in their local areas. People who use hospice services are representatives of the local community who 'own' the hospice. The aim of user involvement is to empower the voice of these representatives so that they can have a meaningful and valuable input into the hospice as an organisation. The challenge of user involvement is in finding ways in which we can hear what people have to say about their experience with their hospice. As professionals involved in the organisation, with ideas of our own, do we have an agenda on what we want to listen to, and what we want to hear when it comes to user involvement? If so, how do we manage this in order to empower and maximise the user voice? How do we manage the potential threat of further sharing responsibility for the organisation with the people who use the services the organisation offers? The most significant common element in both palliative care and creativity is that it values the person in a holistic way. Perhaps creativity can be understood to tell the story of the organisation as it continues on its journey, valuing all ideas and input, so that user involvement can be a fulfilling experience.

User involvement and creativity: a meeting of minds?

Is it possible to have a meeting of minds between user involvement and creativity? This is a question with which I have challenged myself when I became aware of my assumptions, as outlined above, regarding the separate entities of user involvement and creativity. I started to see some potential connections between the two and to feel some excitement about the possibilities that might arise as a result. The connections that arose in my thinking are summarised here.

▓ Process can determine outcome. In creative expression, the process of 'telling the story' has therapeutic value. I began to see that the process of unravelling and expressing a personal story might have similarities to the process a user group might undergo in exploring their experiences with the service, through the conversation and discussion that would occur.

▓ A valuable aspect of creativity is that it validates the stories that people express, and it privileges the meanings of the storyteller in an individual way. If the storyteller is embodied in a user group, validation can occur at a wider level by encouraging contributions to the hospice story by the people who use the hospice.

▓ Creativity and user involvement share the provision of a forum within a hospice setting where an individual or a group of individuals can use their creativity to express something important to them. This could be about capturing and recording the significant moments in a life and exploring that significance in the present and future. This could also lend itself to an expression of views to inform the organisation.

▓ Creativity promotes and empowers individuals and honours the need for honesty in the emotional impact of life with a life-threatening illness, with a view to the creation of something that takes insight from the past in order to inform the future. In a group setting, the undertaking of a project can be a collaborative success with pride extending throughout the group. In a group setting, this could be interpreted as the influence that the group could have in collaborating about the future of the hospice.

▓ People who live with a life-threatening illness (either within their body or within their family) co-exist with degrees of uncertainty. Such uncertainty has an inevitable impact on the experience of family members, and also becomes a facet of functioning with the hospice as an organisation. There is a need to embrace uncertainty and to provide an environment within which people feel an element of safety with uncertainty. In the implementation of both creative projects and user groups, there are no clearly predictable outcomes. Difficulties could arise, and these need to be accommodated and supported within the collaborative journey of the individuals who receive care from the hospice and those who provide that care.

▓ One must acknowledge the reality of organisational fear. There is something potentially scary about embracing creativity, and user involvement, as ways of working when there is no real clarity in the outcomes for people or the organisation in either specific or in general terms. Creativity represents the individual. The embrace of creativity as a hospice is an uncertain journey, reflecting the experience of the people for whom we care. The embrace of user involvement can be understood along similar lines.

▓ Both creativity and user involvement imply some form of empowerment. A commitment to empowering the user voice is an acknowledgement that power needs to be shared. This may be a loss to elements within an organisation that might perceive that they are losing power. The validation that comes with creativity raises the position of empowerment for service users, as a product of the experience. Empowering people means sharing responsibilities and taking a new position in relation to them. Is user involvement a lip service exercise or does it have a real future in informing service?

▓ It is important to continue to see Hospice as a 'Movement'. This implies the normality of change, as a movement should continue to evolve. In order to stay true to core values whilst also moving, creativity and user involvement are potentially powerful voices.

My processes of thinking and unravelling my views about the connections between creativity and user involvement occurred surprisingly quickly for me, so that the connections now appear obvious and I wonder why they had not occurred to me earlier. The position of 'voice' and 'identity' as common elements in thinking about creativity and user involvement will now be discussed.

Voice and identity

The two clear features of 'voice' and 'identity' that are shared by creativity and user involvement can be explored further here. I will comment on these two common features in turn, and look at how they relate to creativity and user involvement.

The Cambridge English dictionary defines 'voice' as follows:

- an expression of opinion
- an important quality or opinion which someone expresses, or the person who is able to express it
- to say what you think about a particular subject, especially to express a doubt, complaint, etc. that you have about it.

Within these definitions, 'expression' is central to the understanding of the meaning of 'voice'. It is important to consider how voice and expression are heard, as well as how they are delivered. In the context of life with a life-threatening illness, it is likely that voice and expression are delivered, and understood, in varied verbal and non-verbal ways. It is likely that basic functioning requires communication in different ways as people adapt to the presence of a life-threatening illness in their life. Palliative care embraces the central idea of 'total pain' and accepts that pain can be experienced and communicated physically, socially, financially, spiritually and psychologically. Creativity exists within the principles of palliative care, which is reflected by the idea that total pain can be honoured as an individual experience as outlined above. The acceptance of the position of 'total pain' enables creativity to have a central role in how people's voices are heard within hospice care. If pain can be more than physical, voice can be more than something that is physically 'heard'. Rather, voice can also be something that is seen, sensed, touched, intuited. The 'hearing' and understanding of voice can be relative to the recipient. It is important that the recipient values the voice and the expression of the voice, in order to value the person who 'voices'. In terms of user involvement in my case, the recipient is the hospice as an organisation. The organisation has a commitment to genuinely hear the voice of service users to inform hospice service and development and to include the user group as a part of the organisation. Voice, within a user group, can be a collective expression from a number of individuals with something to say. Creativity can work with the user group by valuing them as individual and as collective voices, and enabling them to embrace different ways in which they can deliver their voice to inform the development of the hospice as a local charity, and as a national and international movement.

The Cambridge English dictionary defines 'identity' as follows:

> who a person is, or the qualities of a person or group which make them different from others.

Identity is fundamental to who we are as human beings. It should be something that we can define as individuals as we grow, evolve and adapt in our lives. It should be something that is very personal to the individual. However, people who use a service are identified by that service in a way that makes a clear role within which people function in certain environments and situations. For example, commercial business might identify people who use their services as 'consumers' or 'customers'. Legal companies might use the word 'client' to describe the people who use the service they provide. Within a hospital setting, people are described as 'patients'. The word 'patient' is closely related to illness, as the description is determined by the experience of being an ill person in some way, and needing to be made better. The primary role and function people have in being identified as a patient in a hospital setting is in the presentation of their physical body in order that a medical intervention is done to it. Within a hospice, under the defining principles of holistic care, we welcome more than the physical being. Therefore, the 'patient' description is limited and might undermine the potential for how a person adapts to their opportunities to present their holistic 'self' in the hospice environment. One could argue that the label of 'patient' is inherently negative in that it requires a flaw in the physical being to exist in order to merit the description. Hospices should embrace and honour the person's own ideas about their identity within the hospice setting. It is only then that user involvement and user groups can be truly valuable to the evolution of holistic care. Creativity can enable the holistic identity to evolve, and to contribute to user involvement.

As a hospice social worker, I have shared my journey of making sense of the relationship between creativity and user involvement. What seemed to me to be two areas that were worlds apart became meaningful to each other in my mind as I was invited to think about how they would work together. As we move towards the development of creativity and user involvement, I hope that we can develop this relationship in practice as well as in theory. I remarked at the beginning of this chapter some of my anxieties about user involvement and how to move it forward. I now find myself at the bottom of a hill I am excited to climb.

Part 2: the hands project

David Alcock

As a new member of staff at the hospice, employed to develop and deliver a creative programme, I have been asked to discuss how creativity will be used in this environment. Being a newcomer to the field of palliative care I am currently exploring methods in which creativity can be effectively applied.

The creative programme is at its very early stages of development and the project I describe has just been introduced to the hospice. To demonstrate how the project is developing, I use examples of people's work and their responses to it, and talk about how that response has driven the direction of the work.

Project outline

This project uses people's own hands as a starting point for creative projects. Initially photographs and computer scans are made of the hands. There are sometimes difficulties due to people's illnesses. So making sure everyone is included is one of the big challenges. The benefit of starting with a hand is that it is relatively simple for almost everyone to take part. All we need to do is place our hand on a scanner for a few seconds and involvement is immediate. It works as a good icebreaker too, creating a platform for conversation. Because the process is very fast and the hand image can be viewed on the screen immediately, it stimulates lots of response from the participant. People are generally fascinated to view their own hand in this way. Reactions are very varied, from the humorous to the emotional, so this is where the creative process can begin. By picking up on the person's reactions to the image we can start to develop ideas

The hand image will ultimately form part of a collaborative piece; everybody's hand will eventually be printed and combined into a single piece of work. The great thing is that, at this point, people are already making suggestions for how the piece should look. For example, somebody immediately held their hands up, linked their thumbs together and graphically demonstrated how people's hands could be linked into a circle formation. This is a good example of a person who is expressing a strong response to creative input. The aim then is for projects like these to continue to create opportunities for individuals to express themselves, creating a space that allows people's voices to be heard, where they are enabled to present their feelings and thoughts in a format that is suited to their needs.

Case studies

The examples below are real, only the names have changed. I purposely haven't gone into any detail regarding the person's condition. As a non-clinical member of staff I have limited understanding of the nature of people's conditions and I try not to ask too many questions about this, in order to maintain relationships on a level footing. These two cases demonstrate how a common starting point – the hand – can take very different directions depending on the participant.

Example 1: Hannah's framed hand

Hannah, a weekly visitor to the day unit contributed to the hands project by scanning her hand in. She was quite frail, so at this point we decided to leave the work at that stage, with a view to developing it later if an opportunity arose. Eventually Hannah came in for respite. She spent most of her time in her room, so I thought this would be a good time to engage her in some form of activity. We discussed what we could do with the image of the hand, and we soon came up with the simple idea of printing it off and making a frame for it. Hannah wanted to personalise it by decorating it with her name. The end product was very simple yet also moving and powerful. It didn't take us long to achieve results, giving Hannah real ownership over the activity. Hannah proudly placed the piece in her room so visitors could see what had been made. After the completion of Hannah's respite, she soon returned to her regular day unit visits. I enquired into what had happened to the piece of work and she was thrilled to tell me. Her granddaughter had seen it and wanted to take it home. Hannah was delighted to be able to give the piece as an appreciated gift. Finally there was a nice twist to the tale. Hannah's granddaughter had developed the piece to a further level by adding a calendar to it so that she could go to her gran's hand every day. Hannah had produced, with pride, something that was very much her own, and she had seen the real meaning that it had for another person (her granddaughter). This is a case where a simple, accessible and achievable activity can lead to some valuable and meaningful outcomes.

Example 2: Rachel's photo montage

Rachel scanned her hand, and whilst doing this it gave me the opportunity to get to know Rachel. It turned out that family was very important to her, so I asked if she would like to bring some photographs in to show me. We discussed whether we could find a way of combining them with the image of her hand. Next week Rachel had a selection of photographs ready to show me, mostly of holidays and family. We spent a while discussing the photographs, Rachel filling me in on the family members and holidays, talking of happy times. I offered to scan them into the computer so that we could sit back and enjoy them in a slide show format. At this point we decided to come up with a sentence that represented each of the photographs. Many of these would be purely descriptive titles, but others were more emotive and poetic. Snapshots pulled from a conversation, one example being 'A Different Kind of Beauty'. This very poetic sentence came from Rachel looking at a beautiful scene of a holiday landscape, and talking about the attractions that landscapes in other countries hold. Once we completed this process we decided to put the photographs, hand image and text together as a large montage, which was finally printed and framed.

As I write this, the project continues to evolve. Rachel highlighted two of her favourite images from the collection of photographs, I then reproduced this image in the form of a simple line drawing. We decided to start by building up the image through collage, something that Rachel could comfortably participate in, even if she takes part through directing me about which colours to use and where to put them. The image stays very much Rachel's own, from selecting the photo to directing the process; she can claim full authorship of the work. Once this piece is complete, others may follow, or she might feel that she has said all she wanted to say. In either way Rachel has been actively involved in a creative process that has generated lots of positive response.

The initial activity of taking an image of a person's hand can be the start of a creative journey for many but may equally be the beginning and end for others. The latter group may not develop the work further but the key thing is that they have experienced involvement.

Conclusion

To conclude, we would like to comment on the impact of the process of writing this chapter on the development of creativity in user involvement in our hospice. For our first user group we invited patients and carers to give us their views about hospice services and ideas for future development. Following a conversation about their identity, the user group have named themselves The 'TREE' Group. TREE stands for 'Time for Reflection, Expression and Expansion'. There were clear ideas about the impact of growth and discussions about roots and branches. A project is evolving within the day unit to look at how the TREE can reach those people who are unable to come to the group.

Here is a hospice user's impression of the TREE:

Time is for sharing and caring, that we may do what we can
Reflection to think upon, have moments, to see and look forward ... plan
Expression a word to tell each other our ideas, to meet and focus
Expansion develop and grow, spread out as branches and leaves as on our TREE

Helen Monaghan, February 2006

Nuala Cullen BA (Hons) MA DipSW is the Principal Family Support Worker at St Andrew's Hospice in Grimsby. She is trained as a social worker and is in the process of training in Family Therapy. Nuala works primarily in the children's hospice at St Andrew's, but has taken the lead in developing user involvement in the adult hospice.

David Alcock works at St Andrew's Hospice in Grimsby, where he is the Creative Therapy Co-ordinator for adult and children's services. Before this he worked in a variety of settings. These included working as a freelance artist in primary schools, in a community arts group as a Co-ordinator for Creative Projects, and as an Art Tutor in Adult Education. He has also spent a lot of time working in museums – across Lincolnshire, North Yorkshire and Manchester.

CHAPTER 8

No – you *don't* know how we feel

Gillian Chowns, Sue Bussey, Alison Jones, Nick Lunch, *et al*

Introduction

Much of the literature assumes that the 'users' are adults. However, children are also users of palliative care services and this chapter describes an innovative way of combining a popular artistic medium (video) with work with children dealing with parental illness.

The rationale for this came from our own practice. As specialist palliative care social workers, we believed that children were more competent, aware and articulate than many adults supposed. We were dissatisfied with the lack of research in this area and frustrated at the way children were often marginalised.

Thus was born the idea of the video project – to make a video to help families facing parental illness or death. The fundamental principle was that it should be research *with* children, not research *on, about* or *for* children.[1] We wanted to help children to be heard – to have their voice, their experience and their expertise centre stage. As the Introduction to *Handbook of Action Research* makes clear, it was not about being a 'passive data source … but … being able to contribute … experience, ideas and views in all sorts of ways'(*see* page 1).[1] Groups are a powerful form of user involvement, offering (at their best) support, mutual aid and fun, as well as the serious business of working for change 'in line with service users' rights and needs' (*see* page 2).[1]

One idea, many actors – the story of the project

Gillian Chowns

User involvement values everyone's contribution – rarely does anything depend on one person alone, and our project was no exception. This chapter will model the reality of collaborative work by using a number of 'voices' to tell the story from different perspectives. We hope this will demonstrate that user involvement does not have to be daunting, but that different individuals can contribute varying skills – organisational, artistic, therapeutic and 'lived experience'.

I had suggested making a video with children whose parents were seriously ill. A video would be user-friendly – something that parents could borrow and watch at home, that children could watch on their own or together with the family, that could be replayed at will; the idea of making a video should appeal to youngsters because it was a contemporary, exciting and interactive medium; and I was convinced that what the children might say would have far more impact than professionals' opinions.

Once I had discovered the branch of action research called collaborative inquiry,[2] I realised that this was an approach that gave power to the users, recognised their expertise and actively sought to engineer change. All (!) I needed now was some co-researchers. Two social work colleagues were interested and after preliminary discussions, committed themselves to the work. I then approached a filmmaker, Nick Lunch, from Insight. Here I met the first challenge of collaborative working – Nick wanted to do things differently. I found myself listening, negotiating and shifting my position – precisely the things that user involvement in principle, and our project in practice, requires for a successful outcome. Nick persuaded me to adopt his participatory approach to filming rather than the usual documentary style and he in turn yielded to my conviction that we should keep the focus entirely on the children, rather than involving parents.

Recruiting the children is discussed below, but for the nine children who decided to participate, the idea that they could help other families by telling their story was clearly a powerful motivator.

So began the group. We met weekly for seven sessions, either on a Saturday morning or a Friday afternoon. After each session, the four facilitators, myself, Sue, Alison and Nick, would debrief. We three social workers also met weekly, either to plan the next session or for group supervision. Additionally, e-mails flowed endlessly between us. User involvement is not a cheap or quick option; it needs careful planning before, and time for reflection after the actual user sessions.

As is always the case in palliative care, we ran out of time. Just as our clients face the knowledge that time is short, so we struggled with this. We planned for six sessions, but provisionally pencilled in a seventh, which we inevitably needed. At the children's request, we extended the later Saturday sessions from two and a half hours to an exhausting four.

Ideally, the young people would have been fully involved in the editing process. However, this was impossible; the process was extremely lengthy, laborious and skilled, and all the users were in school full-time. So, following a review of the material by the adults, Nick produced a first draft from the footage to which the children had already given consent for use. We also had many hours of footage recorded by our 'process' camera, which had been quietly recording throughout each of the seven sessions. This was primarily for my own research purposes, and not for public use, but with the children's agreement, we were able to include just a little of this material. Our younger co-researchers then critiqued this first draft (with brutal honesty!) and sent it back for further revisions before finally approving it.

At the public launch of the video, one youngster introduced the project, others spoke about particular aspects, and after the showing of the film, they all took questions from the audience. In the year following, we continued this policy of collaboratively disseminating the work, with several of the youngsters speaking at both local and national conferences.

Catching the vision

Sue Bussey

Planning a children's group, particularly one that involves painful and sensitive issues, and where the situation for individual members can change dramatically at any time, feels seriously problematic. Add into the equation a plan to make a video with the group which will be for public consumption, and the hurdles are likely to feel insurmountable. They certainly did for me when Gillian began talking about this project at least a year before it actually took place. Although wanting to be supportive, I was sceptical that it would ever be possible because of a whole variety of problems: engaging a viable group; finding sufficient time; overcoming the issues of consent and confidentiality; getting funding; finding a suitable venue; coping with the group if one of the parents dies; and, finally, producing a suitably professional product when I, for one, knew absolutely nothing about video. Talking to children about difficult issues was the least of my worries, given that it was my daily work within a palliative care team, but the practicalities of this project seemed impossibly complex.

The families we approached about the project indicated that they were at a similar point, namely enthusiastic and interested but with some concerns about privacy and distress for children and patients. For a couple of families these concerns meant that they eventually decided not to take part in the project. We began recruiting children for the project by approaching those children with whom we were already working, as well as asking other palliative care professionals to suggest names. We then held an open meeting for families to explain the project in greater detail. This was a crucial stage; user involvement is a sound idea, but the approach to gathering a group can make or break it. At the introductory meeting, the children had a chance to meet each other and also to handle the video camera and equipment. The emphasis was on it being their project – *they* would decide what themes to cover and how to address them; *they* could choose whether to appear in front of camera or whether to be the operator; and, crucially, *they*, not the adults, would approve or reject the footage.

It seems likely that those who did take part were influenced by a number of factors. Some were already receiving support from the palliative care services and so were perhaps realistic about the illness and open to professional input, willing to trust us and take risks with us. For example, at the open meeting were a 15–year-old boy and his mother. He was confronted with a group of younger girls, two of whom spent much of the meeting whispering and giggling together. He watched the proceedings with deepening horror and afterwards was very reluctant to continue. However, his mother felt a strong commitment to the project and both he and she had a good personal relationship with one of the workers, and so he was persuaded by her to give it a try. He became a highly significant member of the group, making extremely helpful contributions, both to the video itself, within the group, and also in the dissemination of the work afterwards. In a piece he wrote for presentation to a professional conference, he said,

> When I was asked to do this video I was a bit apprehensive because I was the oldest one there and I didn't know anyone, but I realised that no one really knew anyone, and we were all in a similar situation. After the sixth week these people I didn't know became my friends and people who I could relate to.

He clearly did not feel that he had been coerced, and in the evaluation questionnaires that the children completed all said that it was their own decision to attend; seven also said they came because they wanted to help others, and seven said that it was because they wanted a chance to say what they thought.

To quote a young person who moved from initial doubt to full participation in the project:

This experience has affected my life as it made me realise there are others in my unique situation, and I hope other children and young adults benefit from our own experiences as told through the video ... There were a lot of personal issues raised ... and at first I was unsure, but after watching the final video I realised how much it could help others and my concerns went about the video being released into the general public.

Working collaboratively – principles, pitfalls and positives

Gillian Chowns

As Sue has indicated, having a vision and turning it into reality are two different things. *Wanting* the children to be fully involved rather than simply serving as a glorified focus group was not enough – we needed to think carefully about how we could *genuinely* share power with young people who, in family or school, were usually in a dependent role.

At the open meeting referred to earlier, we had tried to model our respect for them as potential partners in two key ways – by giving them, literally, hands-on experience of the video camera, a very expensive and complicated piece of equipment; and by always directing our explanations to them rather than their parents. Thus the message was 'This is your project, and you make the decisions; it is you who are the most important.'

After recruitment comes retention, a difficult issue for many user projects, as well-attended sessions dwindle into a gathering of the faithful few. In our first meeting our intention was to establish collaborative working as quickly as possible, and also to begin to shift the balance of power towards the children.

For example: when everyone was asked to write down their worries about the project, anonymously, and post them in a Worry Box (see Alison's comments later) the adults joined in, acknowledging that they were equally as vulnerable as the children. Also, everyone was asked to film another group member introducing themselves, and when the adults revealed considerable incompetence in operating the camera, this proved very reassuring for the children!

These exercises modelled the adults' identification of themselves as involved collaborators and colleagues rather than detached, powerful leaders. Of course, we could not abrogate all responsibilities as adults and facilitators, but in this first session we needed to establish the principle that the children were in charge of key aspects. The question of refreshments might seem a small matter, but was an excellent opportunity to begin that transfer of power to the users. An adult facilitator explained that it was up to them to choose what they wanted. This provoked plenty of discussion, with the youngsters confidently making suggestions, arguing their case, identifying the practical problems of someone else's idea and finally coming to some sort of consensus, with just a little help from the facilitating adult.

The final task of the first session was to brainstorm the themes they wanted to research for the video. The ideas flowed thick and fast with the children clearly deeply engaged and passionate about what they wanted to explore. The adults had not suggested a single idea and vetoed none that were offered, but valued everyone's contribution. The agenda for the project was set – and it was clearly the children's.

However, user involvement is not without its difficulties. Time-keeping, staying focused, and respecting different viewpoints, were all challenges present in the video project, as much as in an adult user group. Sharing power with young people was often a challenge for the adults, and the *organisation* (as opposed to the experience) of the painting session, was an example of this.

All the children were keen on the idea of painting their emotions and it was suggested we did this in the third session. I was doubtful. It was a Friday after-school session of only 90 minutes and I felt that, given all the other things that had to fit into it, we would not have enough time to do justice to the painting activity. But neither my adult nor my younger colleagues saw this as a problem. Should I go with the users' choice or should I move into leader mode, claim the privilege of experience (that painting sessions always take longer than you think!) and delay it to a Saturday session?

Reluctantly faithful to the principles of collaborative inquiry and respecting the voice of the child, I agreed to the painting plan. The following Friday was frantically busy and both the painting of the pictures and the explanations of their meaning to camera were extremely rushed. We missed an opportunity for richer and deeper discussion – but we still got some good footage, the painting was therapeutic and the children felt more in charge than if their wishes had been overridden.

Learning to work collaboratively

Alison Jones

Although three of us had worked together on projects before, the four of us worked for three different organisations. We anticipated initially a leadership of two plus one extra for emergencies, but by the time we were committed to the project we all wanted full involvement. By then our camera expert explained his wish to be fully involved using participatory video principles. How would we manage with four leaders? Co-leadership had become the norm in group work practice.[3] Could the group feel safe with so many chiefs?

As we were unsure how we would blend our individual styles we met together for an opportunity to examine this. We spent a day discussing the project. We completed an exercise which demanded a certain level of honesty[4] and this enabled us to share our concerns and begin to develop trust in each other. We were four very different people – three middle-aged women, one young male. Three of us brought experience of working in the palliative care field, one came with camera skills.

We decided to share tasks and rotate the leadership, even to sharing the responsibility for buying the food each week. We learnt to communicate our concerns openly at our weekly debrief. We were always fighting against time and initially felt resentment if someone else's slot impinged our own. For me this waned when I realised that the group process was beginning to work, around the same time as Gillian felt the frustration of the time-limited art session!

In their evaluation, the group members were not deterred by having so many adults, but enjoyed the opportunity to relate to each of us.

Effective collaboration required energy, awareness of, and sensitivity to each other. It thus provided a richness of experience which enhanced the whole group.

Working with children and young people

Sue Bussey

Groupwork with vulnerable young people raises ethical issues which need to be considered by all involved. Because it was also a research project, the video project had already been approved by the local ethics committee, but a continuing concern to us as social workers was the fact that this video would be in the public domain, and so confidentiality could be compromised. Clear prior consent had to be obtained from both children and adults, and decisions made about how much personal information to disclose when filming. This careful protection of privacy had to continue beyond the final group session, for example at the public launch of the video, when members of the press were present.

There were also practical problems to overcome, such as parents getting the children to the venue, sometimes immediately after school on busy Friday evenings. We did occasionally have to resort to helping out with transport; obviously volunteer drivers have to be vetted and insured. Those young people with their busy academic and social lives had to give up some other activities up for the duration of the group. Adding a sick parent into the equation complicates what one can ask of families. Fears about the vulnerability of the children could have paralysed us and prevented us from even starting the work, and was one of the reasons we made the decision to run the group in an intensive way. One mother did enter the final phase of her illness during the course of the group, but by striving to manage distressing situations openly and sensitively we demonstrated to the young people that we recognised the impact of these events on their lives and the belief that they would be able to manage and survive them. In this way we saw the group as supporting and building on their resilience and coping strategies.

There is also the added complication of working with and coping with a wide range of ages, backgrounds, interests, and behaviours. One child (or adult) can completely disrupt a group, so it is important to think about how to manage different needs and behaviours. A basic knowledge of groupwork theory is helpful[4] but also it is useful to look at the behaviour of the young people in the light of attachment theory.[5] Of course there were times when we struggled to know how to handle situations. Occasionally the behaviour of one child would irritate others, or another would be particularly demanding of adult attention; given that our group philosophy was to maintain mutual respect and self-determination, we hesitated to adopt an authoritarian approach. As Alison indicated earlier, we were initially concerned that our group would be 'top-heavy' with adults; however, we actually found that at times we needed the four of us to enable the group to function smoothly, particularly when we split into smaller groupings or one child needed some individual attention. There were times, also, when we were able to step back and simply observe them working together on a task. However, it did involve us in a large amount of planning, de-briefing and other communications in between each session, which was probably the key to their smooth operation on the day. We have taken this as an important lesson for subsequent groups, always erring on the side of over-staffing and careful preparation.

Subsequent groups

In group meetings that we have organised for other children since making the video, we have provided a mixture of activities that have included outings for recreation and social contact, alternating with meetings that have allowed more reflection and discussion. We have used the video camera to elicit children's feelings and opinions and have also used artwork and play to facilitate expression of feelings. As it is difficult for children to find time and make travel arrangements during term times we have used a newsletter to create a sense of membership, and then have met face-to-face during school holidays. Any group within palliative care has to confront the issue of change through bereavement, and our pool of children eligible for group membership is constantly changing. Our original video group was always intended to be a closed, time-limited group, but our current group is more open. Development of this work continues to be tentative and cautious, but the making of this video has inspired us to continue to be creative in our work to support children and young people facing likely bereavement.

Participatory video

Nick Lunch

We're not video experts, but we do know what we're talking about.

The comment above came from Rachel, an 11-year-old participant in the project, who clearly understood the value of this video for others facing a similar situation. As a practitioner of Participatory Video (PV) I believe it underlies the fundamental essence of this process: PV is a powerful way to develop the participants' control over the project. The first steps of any PV project I facilitate are concerned with developing confidence and trust in each group member. Empowerment of the individual comes through working as a group together to overcome shyness and lack of self-esteem; and through the instrument of a video camera, self-esteem increases as participants transfer their knowledge and experience to others. A PV message comes across in the participants' own words; they are in control of how they represent themselves. Rather than develop people's technical ability as videographers or filmmakers, PV is used more as a process to develop confidence and group working skills and take people through a process of change as they realise their abilities and affirm their views and beliefs.

A series of simple games was used to develop filmmaking skills, one of which was 'The Name Game'. Everyone sat in a circle, and each person filmed the person opposite, who said their name, and something about themselves while the rest of the group listened. Getting the participants to handle and use the camera in an uncomplicated way is very important right at the start. I showed one person the basics: how to hold the camera, how to record and pause, how to frame the subject in the viewfinder. The camera was passed around the circle with each child showing the next how the camera functioned. The less 'teaching' by the facilitator, the better! I then used the Video Comic Strip activity to challenge the group to work together to plan and film a short sketch about someone slipping on a discarded banana skin. We drew a grid of nine squares on paper as a cartoon strip. Changing the dynamic here from sitting in a circle on chairs to getting on the floor around a large sheet of paper, a shared canvas, injected new energy and mixed the group up. Each person was asked to draw in one box what they wanted to see through the lens and they then directed that shot in the story. They could choose whether to appear as actors in the film but everyone had to direct and shoot a five second clip. To keep things simple at this early stage the clips were frozen images (stills) and silent. This activity aimed to practise the different shot types introduced by the facilitator to learn how to tell a story with pictures. But just as important was helping individuals to develop group working skills and respect for one another, and encouraging them to articulate a choice and achieve a collective, creative endeavour.

Letting go of control, the facilitator's challenge is then to maintain a balance between the groups' ever-changing needs (whether it is a need for a sense of direction, for 'results', or a need for space to redefine the purpose of the project) and the overall task. Flexibility is the key! One must be prepared to change a planned activity at a moment's notice. The process must stay fluid to meet everyone's needs but at the same time there must be a sense of it going somewhere. I found working with the other facilitators was very helpful and inspiring both from the perspective of developing an overall vision and maintaining a rigorous participative methodology. But we were also able to share ideas for non-video type activities that considerably enhanced the process and brought out rich material for the film.

Two techniques I find helpful to inject creative energy into the group decision-making process are 'Think and Listens' and Margolis Wheels.[3] For the former we had groups of two and three sitting together in a quiet corner. Each person was given a minute to think aloud without interruption on a given topic with their partner simply listening. One of the children exercised her right to sit in silence for the duration of her minute. This exercise enabled everyone to get time to prepare their thoughts and ideas before sharing with the wider group (and camera). The Margolis Wheel activity was set up with chairs in the centre, facing outwards. An outer circle of chairs faced inwards so that pairs could discuss an issue and then those in the outer circle moved round to find a new partner for a new topic. This created a dynamic flow of ideas, and worked well to inject energy and allow intimate sharing of personal experience before the brainstorm on 'Tips for Teachers and Points for Parents' sections of the film.

PV should be an experiential learning process. The ability of the video format to replay footage almost instantaneously using the playback function creates a lively feedback loop and serves to reflect back 'our reality'. Watching back footage is an intimate group experience, sharing perceptions and truths, and our playback sessions enabled the group to act as their own teachers, deciding what worked well and what needed improvement.

In some cases playback caused some members of the group to redo an interview, or to suggest we use a discussion captured on the process camera instead as it was deemed 'more natural'. With this group it also acted as a catalyst and generator of energy for the next stage in the process. It may also have encouraged some members to record their own 'video diaries'. Although not everyone in the group was keen on speaking directly to camera in this way, those that chose to do so used the opportunity to good effect. In one case, a child asked her sibling to prompt her with some questions initially; in another, I simply set up the camera in a separate room, and whoever wanted to record a video diary was able to do so in complete privacy.

PV brings everyone to the same level. Hierarchies that exist outside the workshop space tend to disintegrate. The participants are constantly changing roles, from camera operator to subject, from director to actor and the dynamics of power are constantly shifting. The footage captured, even the created 'product', is truly a joint endeavour and as such demands joint ownership and joint responsibility.

Tools for the job, activities and use of creativity

Alison Jones

Our (adult) aims for the group were to make a video, and hopefully to provide a therapeutic environment for children whose parents were seriously ill.

Our main constraining factor was the constant struggle against time, arguably mirroring the families' own dilemmas of living with uncertainty. How were we to facilitate a safe environment to enable a video to be made in a relatively short time? We needed it to be a collaborative experience, and a balance between action and reflection. Armchair theorising would not produce a video!

As adults we had no personal expertise of being a child with a seriously ill parent. We did have specialist knowledge from working in the field of palliative care, and we were able to offer suggestions, and techniques for identifying children's experience.

We began by addressing the power imbalance of the group by rotating the leadership between the adults hoping that the children might lead when they felt comfortable (which they did in a later exercise). We shared the tasks by allocation, even the tea breaks. I wonder now, whether having four adults present actually enabled the idea of power sharing, modelling no specific controller, whilst still having leadership and safety. We attempted to encourage them to 'name' the group, hoping this would promote group ownership, but this idea did not inspire them. We can only assume that the making of the video was focus enough – and indeed, they responded with enthusiasm from the outset to the games, some of which Nick has described, which helped them to learn techniques and acquire confidence prior to filming their own ideas.

Icebreaking
Various activities were used, with an initial quiz game proving most successful. (A sheet of paper was divided into squares, rather like a Bingo card. Each square contained a light-hearted question which could be tailored to the group members, for example 'Who has a pet cat?' or 'Who likes Brussels sprouts?' The task was to put a name beside each question, and thus get people talking to each other. A completed sheet wins.)

As mentioned earlier, we also introduced 'worry cards'. Children could write their worries on these blank cards at any time and post them in a colourful box. The (anonymous) contents would be read out each week. Children shared concerns such as 'I'm worried about seeing myself on TV' and 'I'm taking stress out on others at the moment – how can I stop?' and these were discussed within the group.

Ground rules and planning the programme
A 'quick think' was used for both. Although the exercises were facilitated by an adult, the children themselves planned the programme to include ideas they had identified – the use of information; life outside cancer; mixed emotions; telling the sick person what is bothering you; teachers not to feel sorry for you etc.

Ground rules included 'You can laugh with me but not at me' and these rules and plans were written up and a copy given to each person. (We provided coloured files for every child and each week copies of plans and reviews were typed up and distributed.) The 'quick think' and ground rules were put on display at each session to help us focus.

Regular review time
Each week we began with the same activity. Using post-it stickers we wrote down something good from the previous week and something difficult, with a child volunteering to read out the resulting lists. Everyone engaged well with this process and we found it useful for those who had missed a week, as it enabled them to also share what they had done. For example, one family missed a session because their father had been in hospital; the post-its enabled them to share this information with, and acknowledge the difficulty to, the group. The feedback on what had worked well and what had been less successful was also invaluable for the adult facilitators.

Use of art
The art activity was led by one of the older girls. A 'quick think' again enabled them to explore their chosen topic, 'Emotions felt when a parent has cancer' and each child then

chose an emotion and painted what they felt. Although 'Art' was the concept, it was interpreted differently by each young person. One chose the feeling 'confusion' and wrote a page full of words associated with her feelings around this. She had not previously spoken openly in the group but was clear and moving in her explanation of her work to camera. Another younger member drew a large face with a huge open mouth. One of the group commented that she thought it looked like a scream. He did not have any words to offer, but when asked when he felt afraid or wanting to scream, he replied in a very uncharacteristic quiet voice 'When Mummy is not well'. Again, this was the first time that this very active child had acknowledged why we were together. At this point, I began to relax, realising that the group were genuinely working together. At times their ability to multi-task, eat crisps, talk, move about, and yet be fully aware of what was happening, was disconcerting!

Workbooks and body mapping

Individual work was done occasionally particularly with the youngest member, who did not always have the same attention span as the others. The workbook 'When someone is seriously ill'[6] provided a vehicle for some moving work which was also on the final video.

One of the parents died just before the last session, and the children in the family chose to do a body map of emotions. A life size body outline was drawn and they coloured their feelings inside the outline, according to where they felt the emotion, and what it was (e.g. sadness, fear etc). This was an activity that needed few words but communicated their feelings powerfully to the others, without embarrassment.

Statements

The children wanted to convey information about their ideas to their teachers and parents and we wanted their comments on what 'experts' in the field had to say.

We printed a number of statements on card such as: 'Children should always be told the truth'[7] and 'Children can often worry that they have caused the parents illness'.[8] A child would choose a card, comment on it and then place it somewhere on the floor between two posts labelled 'agree' and 'disagree'. This engaged the children and facilitated further group discussion.

'Children need honesty and openness and the opportunity to talk', for example, generated much discussion. All agreed with the need to know the truth, but one child was able to say that she preferred not to talk, and therefore enjoyed being with her grandparents who did not force her to talk, as they preferred also to say nothing. She rarely appeared on camera but she was an enthusiastic group member who was happier behind the camera and letting others speak.

Our activities were all enablers to facilitate the group process, which they seemed to do successfully. The children were quick to disregard what they did not want (like the name of the group) and quick to instruct us.

After one meeting, while awaiting their transport, they engaged in a spontaneous game of 'tag' (in the car park!) involving all ages. Their request the following week was for more 'fun', reminding us that, although we had a serious project to complete, they needed to include physical fun. We had our next break time in the garden playing 'ladders' - a challenging activity for some of the middle aged! They were keen for the fun activity to be included in the video to illustrate the point 'that you cannot be sad and distressed all the time'.

Conclusion

Three things stand out clearly from this example of working creatively with young users. First, video was an excellent medium to use. It was contemporary – attractive to the children and 'cool'; it was powerful – effective in getting a message across to viewers; it was immediate – the children were able to review what they had just filmed and get immediate feedback. And equally importantly, participatory video shared the same values as those underpinning the philosophy of user involvement.

Secondly, young people – the co-researchers were aged 7 to 15 – may be more competent, confident and articulate than most adults are willing to recognise. Many professionals focus on children's *vulnerability*, but this project assumed *ability* – and we believe its assumptions were justified.

Thirdly, user involvement is not an easy option; it is hard, skilled work and requires time for planning and reflection as well as action. It is a process more than an event, an attitude more than an activity, and it is slow-growing rather than instant. But its benefits for users, professionals and their organisations may last long after the particular project is complete, and continue to challenge the way we work in palliative care.

As one of our young users said, as she reflected on what she had gained from the group, 'Before, I couldn't actually say that my dad had cancer, in case people might laugh – but now I can, and they don't'.

Acknowledgments

All four co-authors wish to acknowledge Jack, Becky, Rachael, Laura, Megan, Laura, Gemma, Natalie and Ellis who were co-researchers on the video project as well as 'users' of palliative care services; the authors are indebted to them for all that they gave to the project.

Gillian Chowns is a Senior Lecturer in Palliative Care at Oxford Brookes University and a former Specialist Palliative Care Social Worker with the East Berks Macmillan Palliative Care Team. Her career has encompassed all three major statutory agencies – Social Services, the NHS and Education. She has recently completed a doctorate on the subject of children facing the life-threatening illness of a parent. She also has a strong interest in international palliative care.

Sue Bussey is a Specialist Palliative Care Social Worker with the East Berks Macmillan Palliative Care Team, which pioneered specialist pre-bereavement work with children. Sue has worked for both statutory and voluntary social care organisations, including the Lady Hoare Trust and has specialist expertise in working with children with disabilities and chronic or life-limiting illness.

Alison Jones is a former Principal Social Worker with Thames Hospice Care and was instrumental in setting up their Bereavement Service. She is a qualified counsellor and since her retirement has worked as a supervisor and trainer for Cruse Bereavement Care.

Nick Lunch has been an enthusiastic advocate and pioneer of participatory video (PV) techniques for 10 years and is Director of Insight (www.insightshare.org), which has used participatory video with communities and marginalised groups across the globe. He is currently involved in developing the use of PV as an advocacy tool for the United Nations Development Programme's global human rights strategy and working with leading UK research institutes to promote PV as a participatory research tool and instrument for increasing the impact of research findings on policy makers. He has recently edited a handbook on participatory video.[9]

CHAPTER 9

The support group at my shoulder

Lucinda Jarrett and the St Thomas's Hospital Breast Cancer Care Support Group

Introduction

Rosemary Burch, Breast Care Nurse

When I was asked to provide a brief introduction to this chapter I was more than a little daunted; how could I begin to describe the adventure that is the Drop-in Support Group for Women with Early Stage Breast Cancer? It began in March 1992, when three colleagues and I recognised that large numbers of women attending St Thomas's for radiotherapy had no access to any support through their treatment. We decided to experiment, amid some encouragement, but with considerable suspicion that a group might become dangerously out of control. Fourteen years later, the other three have left, but the group has plodded on with largely the same founding principles. We meet for two hours once a week in a wonderful group room with facilities for tea making, and an adjacent complementary therapy room. The setting itself is an informal antidote to the clinical severity of the hospital, and helps to set the tone for relaxed discussion.

It is now well known that every year some 42 000 women will be diagnosed with breast cancer. Most of those will be successfully treated and will resume normal activities after treatment. However, it is also well known that for some, the disease will return, and that every year some women will die of their disease. Although the outlook for breast cancer continues to improve with early detection, increasingly sophisticated diagnostic techniques and therapeutic improvements, for each woman given the diagnosis there is a burden of uncertainty about her future. While many are able to accommodate this with astonishing tolerance, it has long been clear to me that peer group support can be a powerful tool in bringing this about. Talking about difficult experiences, comparing notes about practicalities, exchanging information about the disease, treatments and how to live with it, and perhaps above all, sharing warmth and humour, all contribute to lessening the loneliness of the individual experience, and reducing the anxiety it generates. Breast cancer treatment can sometimes be mutilating, often exhausting, and can undermine body image and a woman's sense of self. As one woman put it, 'I'm flat-chested, bald and knackered, with the energy of a slug, so getting back to normal, whatever that may be, is a bit of a challenge!' But as another quietly commented in response, 'Getting better is a process – you don't get back to your old self as much as find a new and different "normal" that might be stronger than you ever realised.'

Each week, as ten to fifteen women come, usually including one or two newcomers, I am constantly impressed with their resilience in coping with the marathon of treatment and recovery, and with the generosity they demonstrate towards each other.

When Lucinda Jarrett, from Rosetta Life approached us with the idea of doing some creative workshops with any of the women who were able to come an hour earlier, I was delighted, but a little nervous that no one would accept the offer. The eventual results, which included pictures, poems, dance, drama, and an astonishing theatre performance, were overwhelming and exciting, as distress was translated into creativity and given a voice to express both the pain and the cumulative triumphs of this experience.

The support group

Lucinda Jarrett

In a pleasant room looking out over the River Thames with views of the Houses of Parliament and the 'Wheel', the coffee table is set and chairs arranged. The room catches the morning sun and all is ready. People arrive and the conversation increases as they remove their coats, are introduced and offered refreshments. They may know most of the others or may be there for the first time. Someone may arrive with luxury biscuits or a homemade cake. The conversation may range across the responsibilities of the mayor, the difficulties experienced at a child's school, planned holidays. There may be laughter or tears, commiserations or celebrations.

This is not the setting for the average 'coffee morning'. Although the surroundings are comfortable and the view eye catching, one woman, a regular attender, pointed out to me, 'I can't say I've ever thought how beautiful the room is; it does have a nice view of the Houses of Parliament, but it is in a tower block in a hospital full of sick people. The food is good on the ground floor though, and there are shops and a cash machine which are useful. The only reason I would want to go there is to meet other women with breast cancer and get support from them. I can't see myself whiling away time there; I need to get to work.'

For others too, the beauty of the surroundings is the backdrop only to important experiences; the support and the weekly scenes from people's lives which are played out in this room. Here women experience a safe place to talk and listen, to forge a collective voice, if required, or create a strong sense of affirmation. It was this last point which lead me to propose a creative project that would offer to those interested a public platform for their voice. In March 2005 I began working with some of this group: women living with breast cancer. As we worked I became increasingly interested in the group as a whole and what it meant to the women involved.

This chapter looks at the experiences of the whole support group largely in their own words. It looks at the difference between support and voice, between forging the confidence of one's private identity and the assurance of a public voice.

The support group offers women just that: support enabling them to feel confident to be true to themselves at home and in the hospital, or even to themselves and each other. For many the gain in confidence leads them to become better informed and more involved in the delivery of care to them. A creative project within the support group offers a clear and confident identity with which to confront the wider public, a chance to become involved with the formation of a collective representation of how people are living with breast cancer and a chance to make clear statements with a clear voice.

A 'public voice' has a social and political outcome that is not part of the agenda of the support group. Below the women outline some of the reasons for becoming involved in the support group and what is achieved through it. The accounts are drawn from email correspondence, interviews and telephone conversations that I initiated and continued with several of the women of the support group.

Finding support

Anyone, man or woman diagnosed with breast cancer for the first time will experience a range of emotions and be faced with any number of decisions. Through the early stages of acquiring information (some sought, some imposed) those now involved in this support group had been offered information about the group. The information had come either from the breast care nurses directly, or from leaflets or directories of cancer support facilities.

Some attended the group initially for information; others felt isolated or lonely in their experience of treatment. One woman described the anxiety she experienced about the treatment she was being offered and this led her to turn to a place where others might offer advice. Women discussed how comforting and accessible the word 'support' was while they found 'counselling' or 'therapy' difficult and stigmatising. Many have had the benefit of family support which all agreed was invaluable, when available. Others declared that their families had been 'of no support whatsoever, if anything they required support from me'; for some, there is no family. None of the women underestimated the value of an independent support network, appreciating the very real value to be gained from talking with others who have or are going through similar experiences.

Support within the group

The support group creates a place where people can meet, can be themselves without being judged. At the time of writing all regular attendees are women so it is of their experiences we write. Men with breast cancer are welcome and some have attended.

Throughout our conversations 'being myself' was very significant to everyone. This was in fact on two levels. People did not feel that they had to be positive. As one woman put it, 'Often I don't feel like being positive and yet everyone around me feels I am failing them if I am not.' Another agreed, saying, 'Other people often go on about how you must be positive as if being positive affects the course of your illness; according to all the best research, being positive makes no difference to the outcome. These utterances from the ill informed probably make them feel better about what is happening to you but are highly irritating in that they are demanding you feel something you don't.' Yet another said, 'The group is a place where I can feel negative at times without being judged a failure'. And then 'being myself' is also about being really honest and being comfortable with the truth about treatment, outcomes, feelings and the family. 'I feel safe, I can be myself and I won't be judged' was incredibly important.

At another level, leaving behind the roles through which we are identified and possibly constrained in the public arena was equally significant. Mother, nurse, carer, teacher, boss, wife, secretary are all left behind at the door of the room for the support group sessions. Each individual is free to offer only those aspects they want to share. Said one, 'I bring with me more honesty that I have outside the group and am as honest with myself as I am with everyone else'.

Each woman presents herself without the histories of family or private and public identities. Nonetheless the words 'friendship' and 'family' are used in connection with the group which creates for the participants a feeling of belonging, being part of a family. Everyone is welcome as an old friend and the warmth with which people ask each other how they are managing is honest and genuine.

For each woman support is emotional, psychological and can be practical. Essentially the activity of the group is based on finding acceptance and sharing experiences. It is not a site for activism, politics or change. Occasionally the group will welcome a visitor, such as the Chair of the hospital, or collectively support a letter on their behalf. There may be spin offs such as the creative project with which I am involved or the activity of writing this chapter. Individual members of the group may get together to represent their voice elsewhere. For the group itself, finding acceptance is more important than finding a voice. 'It is not a place where we lobby for change or ask for representation, but rather a place for support and that is very different.'

'It is about reassurance as much as anything else. The group provides a holding space for pain but it does not take it away or give me anything to make it better. Sometimes when I leave the group I can sit with the pain slightly more comfortably than before, but not always.' 'Sometimes it can be quite painful to attend, on several occasions people have burst into tears. It is not all joy and rapture. But you know that if you felt as bad and let others see it in the group you would be supported, despite the pain.' 'Sometimes there is something to celebrate; sometimes there is pain to share. I know that the group will do both with me, and I with them.'

Sharing experiences

Those in the support group recognise and value the fact that not everyone has had the same experience. The illness, the treatments, and the individual experience of these will vary. Each woman will have her own story to tell about her diagnosis, and the way it was communicated to her. Each will bring her own previous associations, fears and fantasies which lend meaning to this news. Similarly, tolerance or lack of it for surgery, chemotherapy, radiotherapy or endocrine treatments will fuel much discussion. 'The straw that breaks the camel's back' may vary, and strength and reassurance can be exchanged when this is understood. The women demonstrate a willingness to share their experiences and that of others.

The role of the group facilitator is much valued. In the words of group members – she remembers each individual's name and ensures introductions are carried out. 'Rosemary helps a lot as she ensures that a few people don't dominate and she creates a very good atmosphere where people can contribute. I think that the group would not be as successful without her input.' This description itself emphasises the ownership of the group experienced by the participants.

That ownership is important but the professional support is recognised as essential to the effectiveness of the group. For new members of the group, in particular, the appropriate modelling of the role of the breast care nurse is helpful as is the recognition that permission is given to question and comment. The opportunity to ask about concerns 'in passing', rather than by making an appointment or phoning specifically, is invaluable. The role of the healthcare professional includes the offer of advice or practical help, such as contact with departments, in what can be the somewhat confusing organisation of cancer treatment, and up-to-date comment on any of the myths surrounding cancer which may be raised. On other occasions reassurance that there will be no clinical issue arising from an apparent delay is sufficient. (In fact delay is not a common theme either discussed or indeed experienced amongst these women.) Such support work not only reduces the women's anxiety but also saves NHS resources!

The willingness of members of the group to share experiences within this environment not only enables people to feel supported but often leads to solid practical advice so that people can feel more involved in their medical care. For instance, one woman told the story of a new participant asking, 'Should I have a mastectomy with a reconstruction?' She had felt pressurised into this and wondered if she had any options. Within the group there were those who had had simple mastectomies, others had decided on immediate reconstructions, yet others had wanted to wait for reconstruction. All were able to contribute their experiences including those who had opted for mastectomies without reconstruction. These experiences may include not only the treatment outcomes but information about where further, if necessary, professional advice can be found.

Practical help will also come from others in the group. Some form friendships which impact outside the group, for example, offering practical help with visiting, shopping or more social occasions. Others will research on behalf of the group. One woman found that aqueous cream did the same job as the more expensive vitamin e creams and moisturisers and it was then discovered that it was cheaper over the counter than on prescription. Experiences of handling the symptoms of chemotherapy are exchanged: to shave the head or not to shave the head, what to use as an insect repellent after surgery. Very popular are those with remedies for hot flushes!

Other types of practical issues can be talked through. For example; whether, when and how to return to work. How can they work flexibly to make sure that they maintain their health during a difficult period? What are their legal and employment rights? The support that the women offer each other gives them the confidence, the language and the information to use in the various spheres within which they operate. 'I think that the group tends to support people to stay off work' said one woman, but 'when I first went to it I was already planning to return to work the following Monday and I am really glad I did.' Another described her experience of returning to work supported by the group to the extent that she and a colleague, who had also experienced breast cancer, engaged with their human resources team and offered an informal support group across the large public sector organisation for which they work. In this case, group members were soon asked to offer advice to managers about the 'return to work' process as well as meeting with those who had direct experience of cancer. A more unexpected outcome was the identification of the specific needs of those who had cared for loved ones with cancer.

What do we take away?

'You bring your experience to the group and your support for each other and the group gives you the strength to accept the bits about you that you are unsure about. The inner strength is hard to measure but this is what we take away with us.'

All the women agreed that the support group gave them a place to say what they thought and felt without judgment and that the most significant outcome for them was the confidence this gave them when speaking about their illness and treatment either in confidence to medical professionals or to friends and family.

One woman spoke about how the group became a place that helped to sort out the language for illness beyond the labels of the tabloid press. For her, the issue was the language of the 'fight' and the 'struggle' and how this labelled people as weakened, defeated or conquered by illness. Together the women could find phrases like 'taking responsibility' or 'supporting our issues in our own way'.

Interestingly, one woman reported that after attending the group several times she felt more confident asking questions of her doctor or consultant. In her words, 'I bring the group with me. I carry it at my shoulder into consultations and appointments. It is almost as if the group is at my side whispering in my ear! This may mean that there is a different emphasis to the questions I ask, or a different confidence in my articulation of the questions. I think that, because of my involvement with the group and this increased confidence on my part, I have, on occasion, received a more helpful type of response from healthcare professionals. It seems to give a different weight to my words and perhaps makes it easier for them.' Another retorted, 'What a shame we don't have confidence in our views without the experience of others, but I am afraid the presence of men with white coats, sheaves of files and large machinery seems to disable us.'

Others echoed this feeling of carrying the group with one and talked about speaking more openly of their experiences to friends and family because they felt less isolated and less peculiar. They were able to recognise that their feelings were somehow normalised or made familiar by the experience of the group.

The women also found that their friends and families seemed reassured that they attended the group. Others felt that 'in some cases attendance at the group is likely to worry relatives, as some people may rely on its support more than on their partners, friends and families. I think my mother feels it has had a bad influence on me (along with the Breast Cancer Care Forums) because continuing to take part in support groups encourages you to keep on thinking about breast cancer when perhaps you should have moved on.'

In general friends and family seem to worry less when they know that the support of the group is available. Even unsupportive partners know that the group is part of the routine of the women's lives and know that regular attendance is part of the treatment and healing process. Others have no friends or family and for them the group represents their entire support network.

Perhaps most pertinently, one woman reminded me, 'No support group can deal with the fact that after I had one breast cut off I am left with a chronic condition. The treatments are horrible, particularly mutilating surgery, poisoning chemo and burning cancer causing radiotherapy. Nor do I like the hormone treatment which has been described as chemical castration in a medical article I read; that I should add was not meant for patients' consumption. It would be great if we got cures instead of the drug companies trying to come up with medication to make it a chronic condition. What we really need are more breakthroughs in understanding breast cancer. We are left managing the fall out and that is where the support groups come in.'

Accounts from two women

First account
I first came to the group after my initial chemotherapy session. The day before I had been to the 'Recovery in Motion Day' at Guys Hospital and was reminded by the complementary therapist, that the support group met on Fridays. Rosemary took me into the first session and introduced me to everyone there as it was my first time. I was made very welcome. At the session one member of the group brought up a programme which had been on TV the previous night about someone who was leading a campaign for the use of Herceptin for early stage breast cancer. We had a discussion on treatments which we thought would benefit us and were or weren't available and whether we thought they should be. On some occasions someone will ask a question which also leads to discussion. People join in with the discussion or just listen as they want to do. You sometimes find that your question will be answered even if you have not asked it.

As it was my first session I was offered the chance to have a massage, which was very relaxing. New members to the group are given this opportunity if time permits, or if there are too many newcomers in that session then they will have the first chance on the next occasion they attend the group. Many people come along to every session or as many as they can manage. It is a bit like a club but also like a family as we are all being or have been treated for breast cancer. Our health is sometimes the only thing we talk about especially if there is someone who has a problem.

I asked a question about a dry mouth and a strange taste in my mouth due to my treatment. Other members of the group were able to make suggestions including a mouthwash and buying a tongue scraper to remove some of the fur which was causing me problems.

On another occasion someone raised a problem they were having with money. There is a booklet about financial help which you can get if you have cancer. There weren't any of these leaflets in the room so one woman went downstairs and brought back all of the information which was needed.

Sometimes issues are raised which can be troubling, someone has a recurrence or another problem relating to their cancer or treatment, not all sessions are happy or light-hearted, but on those occasions Rosemary makes sure that we leave the session having given support for that individual but reassured that the same thing may not happen to us. We do know that we can share our problems and will receive help from the group. We support each other and rejoice when there is good news about test results or the end of treatment.

People tend to come along regularly for the length of time that they need support, but even if they come back after quite a long break the group still has a place for them and there seem to be those who remember them apart from Rosemary. We also share parts of our own stories and those of our family life that we want to, but there is no pressure to share more than you want to and we all know each other by our first names only. We don't even share addresses unless we want to. This means that we can tell others exactly what we want and gives a chance to share things with the group which we may not have shared with our families. Our own family may not understand us.

Another role of the group is to provide support of different sorts for the other members. We can help one another by sharing our experiences over everything. Even once the treatment has come to an end, for some people this is the time when they still need to feel that they have support to get their lives back to normal when they return to work or the outside community, or even when we are meeting healthcare professionals because we have had a chance to take views we have all talked about with us away from the session.

Second account
After my radiotherapy finished I felt that my treatment was complete and I thought, 'What now?' I also felt lost and isolated. I believed that I had NOT got rid of the cancer completely. I was invited to St Thomas's Support Group and shared my fears with Rosemary and the group. Their support has enabled me to get through the experience of having three primary cancers in two years. I have been unlucky to have had the cancers but very lucky to have gained some great support and made some very strong friendships.

My experience of the support group
As well as the creative project on which I worked with several members of the support group, about which a whole separate chapter needs to be written, the collaboration on this chapter has raised for me a number of questions and confirmed the value of real

confidence in enabling people with illness to contribute to decisions about their treatment and care in a meaningful way ... not simply by being offered a 'choice' of hospitals.

I have enjoyed the contact I have had with women who are trying to manage their illness, the treatments and their subsequent lives in a constructive way but most importantly 'their way'.

The group offers people a place where the story of each person's cancer was one that found an individual narrative articulated by each person. Through most of my working life I am aiming to identify, with them, opportunities for those seeking a voice. I value the reminder of the enhancing role of 'support'.

CHAPTER 10

The women's group

Suzy Croft and the St John's Hospice Women's Support Group and Francesca Beard

St John's Hospice women's support group

Suzy Croft

Introduction

This is our story of a women's group. We are a group of HIV positive black African women. This is what we think of the group, what we find helpful, what we do and how it makes it possible for us to be more involved in what happens to us and to have more control over our lives. These are our own words. We recorded this discussion then Suzy, who supports the group, put what we said together on paper and we have agreed how we want it to read.

Who we are

First let us tell you something about ourselves. This is how we want to introduce ourselves. These are the issues we want to talk about. We don't want to use our own names. There is too much discrimination. [Editor's note. All names used are pseudonyms.]

Jane: first of all, I was a patient in this hospice. When they told me about the group I thought that would be fine, to go to a place where I could talk about my feelings with people who had the same problem, I thought it was good to know what other people were going through and to share.

Linda: when I first started coming to St John's Hospice it was more men than women and sometimes you were the only woman there, and it was really uncomfortable and it was putting me off. When the women's group was introduced it was really exciting. I've learnt a lot and I've made friends from the women's group. I've talked about things I could never have talked about in the hospice and I've had a chance to express my feelings.

Anne: with me, why I thought I should get involved in the hospice and the women's group was I had a lot of problems going on, so I found that I could at least have someone to talk to here, share my problems and have some of them resolved. And there were so many things, like with the pain I was going through, just getting out of my house, coming to meet other women, other people and access therapies, which was smoothing my pain. And things like the gym, that was helpful.

Elizabeth: when I first came to the hospice there were only two other women. Now since we have started this group it is good to see we can talk one to one with other women, because with most of the day centres they place the emphasis on the needs of the boys, so I am happy when we talk about women. Yes, the men dominate definitely. We need our own privacy as women. Sometimes they need their own privacy as men and we are happy.

Alison: a good thing about the group is that sometimes you think you are going through things on your own and when you come to the group you find that others are going through the same thing, with medication or struggles in a relationship, different kinds of things, so you are not alone. It's quite good to know. We talk about how things are going outside, your life, you share a bit, so you are all right, you know 'it's not just me'.

Pamela: for me I can say I have gained because before I used to be scared, but from going to the women's group I've got strength to go to college without fear. Because of the way I was brought up – in the women's group you find different ages – back home I don't think I could even open my mouth. If I was back home you know I am scared to talk, but here you can talk and say anything you want. You can ask anything you want without fear. Back home it goes by age, so if you see anyone older than you, you can't say anything, you have to be quiet, stay quiet. That's the way I was brought up, but here it is different. I can share my pain.

What we like
Some of us meet outside the women's group. We meet here but we also meet outside, so that is something good.

I quite agree. The women's group has given me strength as well. It's made me realise I am not the only one living with HIV. There are women there who are HIV just like me and there are people who have been on the medication more than I have been and they are looking well and I thank God for that.

Yes there is another lady who comes to the day hospice called Mabel. She is looking very, very nice and young and so it gives me hope. Maybe she is the same age like my mum and she is living well. She always calls me to see how I am.

I think the women's group is very good for us because when you come here you can discuss women's issues. You can't discuss when men are there because they make fun of you.

When we have had people to talk about different issues, that was quite good

Yes having speakers coming in, that is really nice.

Doing new things
The exposure has been good. You have exposed us to so many things, like meeting the woman poet Francesca. That has been one of the best things. Because before we didn't know what it was like to speak in front of people. I have learnt a lot of things. There are so many skills which I have picked up, like even just presenting myself, how to arrange things, how to write things, even things that have helped me plan my future. Now I think 'I can do it', I've got all these talents, it has brought up my talents and it encourages me

to do more – just to think maybe I can write a book or just write poetry and that helped me with my presentation. Like with the way I am studying it has helped me to speak in front of people. It's really brought different things from different angles for me and I don't now feel depressed, I even forget the pain I am going through, that is physical pain. At first with the script [when we were involved in the radio play Francesca wrote] I used to think, 'Do I need to read all this?' But you know when she did the script you look at it and it is so interesting, and then there is the part where you have to sing. So you think of different talents you are capable of.

Meeting Francesca through the women's group has been very interesting for me [too] because she has helped me to find one of my inner parts, which is like expressing myself because I am not really the talking kind. But finding Francesca through the women's group I have learned to write a lot, and through writing I find that I am expressing myself and I am writing things. Even at home right now, I just take a book and start writing and I am filling the day. At the end of my writing I feel like I have spoken to someone and she's taught me how to write poems and to be able to write poems and to write a poem that is very interesting and I find there is so much emotion for me. In the [radio play] script when we were singing the song the words were very emotional – but we got through it anyway. The words were like 'from the water, from the water we come'. It was very simple, but the more we got to sing it, 'from the water' and you think of yourself and how you can be cleansed by pure water. The water is so beautiful and when you drink it. I even wrote a poem about water after that. It was just so touching.

For me it was like miraculous. I was very down at that time but I realised that I could create a poem, read and perform in front of that audience. I felt cheerful.

I lost my dad last week and then I thought I can read a poem about my dad in front of people, because I have done it here. I did it in Nottingham because there are a lot of Kenyan people there, like a ceremony. We had about 1500 people there, just praying. We had a programme [for the event] and I did it.

Getting involved in a discussion about disability
It was interesting being involved in that, because you don't know your rights generally, what you are allowed to do as someone who is disabled, what people expect from you. So when you know what your rights [are] generally, it is more easy for you to discuss what you want to discuss and don't talk about what you don't feel like talking about. Because sometimes when you go for a [job] interview or something like that you feel you need to tell them, but you don't have to. You don't have to discuss everything. If you feel like it, you can tell someone about it but if they are not acting the way they are supposed to you can complain, so that is good.

Before I didn't really know what disability meant. For me disability was someone in a wheel-chair or something like that. So I understand more what it was about, disability. So it can be with cancer or with HIV. I am more confident. Before, when I stopped using the wheel-chair I was a bit ashamed to show my taxi card in case somebody say 'Why you need that, you look healthy!' So after that it felt normal, you know, you don't have to use a stick or wheelchair to be disabled. So I feel more confident and I know a lot of people have the same problem.

What is helpful in the group

I feel I have had a lot of support from the women's group, I have had financial assistance, information about solicitors, I've really learned a lot in the group, in the discussions and I've had support.

I think the lady [who came to speak with us] from the Terrence Higgins Trust was helpful. She spoke about immigration and she talked a lot about what we are entitled to and what our rights were.

It is good here, the rule as well, the rule that you can come and sit with people but you don't discuss what you are here for. I was struggling because I wanted to go to this day centre but I couldn't talk about the thing I am going through. When the women's group started that was really good, because that was OK, we can talk about HIV, without feeling you can't.

That's another thing the women's group has brought us very close, all of us. Because even in the day centre when you find another woman sitting there, you don't know her, we never even used to say 'hi' to each other. We just sit down and watch each other. When the women's group started we all know each other now, and that's very, very good.

We are African, we are used to socialising very easily but you don't forget that in a different place. A lot of people don't know that. Here you know people live by themselves, they don't know about the neighbour, we are used to [it being different]. ·

It was like a stepping stone for me, this group. Of all the groups I go to I prefer this one. This was the first time I had been in a group. When I came here I felt confident, I felt you can talk freely, you can interact. If I can sit here in a group, then I can go somewhere else and attend another group without fear. I like it when I come to the centre [as well] because you can do what you like and people don't mind. You choose who you want to sit with, I think it's all right.

I find people in the women's group very good and friendly.

Support about immigration

It's been very helpful having a support letter for my immigration from here, that has been the most helpful thing. I am very, very happy about it, in case of anything I know there is always someone to turn to. The social workers know about my solicitor so I am happy about that.

And they have promised to help me and I am very grateful.

Speaking on immigration I include the Department of Work and Pensions as well! It all comes in the envelope. It is such a stressful life to lead and reading the letters they write to you, hearing the Home Office, you feel the whole world is falling apart and it is just you alone. And when you come to the women's group you find you are not the only one. You get to ask your friends what their [immigration] status is, and they get to tell you and you go 'oh, OK …' With the DSS [the social workers] have just been so helpful, so much. Without all that I wouldn't have a flat to start with!

There was one of the boys who was talking about his immigration status and a group of the other boys, they were so surprised. 'How did you come here, how did you live?' They had never heard anything about it. But we know about it, what's going on. [The man] is very, very desperate. He had no one to chat with about it, and so I talked to him. He looked very, very desperate. He comes here in the day centre, he had loads of problems. But when he tried to talk about it with the other boys they looked at him as though he had done something wrong. But what I did was I talked to him one to one, so at least he was a bit happier. And I think a lot of other people [who use] the day centre don't know about [the problems you have] with immigration. If you happen to chat about it here, they think we are not normal – an asylum seeker with HIV. So it is good we can talk one to one about what is going on. Because some of the people who go to [other places for people with HIV], some of them have never heard of going to a support group and getting a support letter from the group, and I told him to go the group and ask for a support letter.

Conclusion
We think groups like this are helpful for us in all sorts of ways.

Please, please, please don't stop the women's group!

Working in partnership with the women's group at St John's Hospice

Francesca Beard

I first meet Lucinda Jarrett at a spoken word night in the bar of the Institute of Contemporary Arts. I am just starting out as a performance poet and she has not yet begun her work at Rosetta Life. We talk for hours about poetry and autobiography.

Lucinda contacts me again in January 2004. I have found my feet – and my voice – as a professional poet. My solo show, Chinese Whispers, is semi-autobiographical. Lucinda tells me about the work she does with Rosetta Life and asks if I would be interested in running some workshops for the Rosetta Live Festival. My mother has died unexpectedly three months earlier and I have been thinking a lot about death and life.

Lucinda matches me with a women's group based at St John's Hospice. In St John's Wood, there is a small private hospital where celebrity mums go to have their babies. At the back of this relaxed and expensive building is St John's Hospice, a charitable organisation funded by the trustees of the hospital. Every second Monday of the month, a small group of women meet for lunch and conversation. These women come from all over London. They are mostly originally from the continent of Africa – Uganda, Kenya, Cote D'Ivoire, Zambia, Tanzania … it's a diverse group of mature students, housewives, an accountant, an actress. Some are unemployed. Some have children – in London or back 'home'. There's one other thing they have in common – they all live with HIV.

Lucinda takes me to meet Suzy and Katherine, the social workers who work with the group. Suzy is friendly but forthright – she makes no bones about telling me that she is there to support and protect the women and that these workshops must be approached with consideration for each individual's privacy and emotional needs. If anyone from the group does not feel comfortable with the workshops, then the project cannot go ahead. She stresses that disclosure is a huge issue around HIV. Some of the women have not told their own children that they are positive. They will not necessarily want to be pouring out their 'truth' in poetic form. It is scary to be confronted with the reality of leading these workshops, but I am glad Suzy has been so clear. Katherine is gentle and empathetic – she suggests that the ladies might not want to focus on death, but rather life. We all think this is a good plan.

At the next planning meeting, we find that Suzy and Katherine, their reservations notwithstanding, are prepared to work incredibly hard to ensure the best possible results for the workshops. We agree that, subject to the willingness of the group, I am to lead four poetry workshops, focusing on exploring the individual 'voice' and turning autobiography into fiction. The workshops will focus on the individual women rather than their disease. If these workshops go well, there is a possibility of running two more, taking the work to performance. The women's group could then take part in a night at the Riverside Studios, presenting their poetry. We all acknowledge that this is probably unlikely to happen, due to the particular issues surrounding HIV.

I meet with the women's group on Monday 10 May. The ladies are witty, hospitable and welcoming. They are also very courteous. In Britain, people are generally quite comfortable with being rude to protect their self-interest. I perceive that there might be a cultural difference at work – I have a deeper appreciation of Suzy and Katherine's protectiveness to this group. I imagine that these African women would hate to hurt my feelings to the extent that they might be prepared to put up with a workshop situation they did not enjoy, rather than say anything negative. I feel OK about this as Suzy and Katherine are participating in the group and I don't have any doubt that they will tell me if it isn't going to work. I am glad they are there as it enables me to relax and do my job.

In the first workshop, I talk about what I do and where I come from. I speak about my childhood in Penang and my feelings of homesickness when I left Malaysia, all my friends and family, to come to school in England. I talk about hating the cold and the food. And I talk about what I love about the UK – the relative freedoms, the sense of humour, the diversity of London. We go round the circle and hear stories of courage and exile and life and loss. We hear about favourite colours and food and animals; first memories and words, our favourite thing about London and what we hate about it, what we would do if we were Prime Minister, what we dream about. We run out of time.

Thereafter, we meet on 17 May, and on all four Mondays in June. Suzy and Katherine are very much part of the workshops. I consult with them on the content of each one and we talk during the week about how it went. They pick up on things I miss and they also contribute creatively. They are wonderful.

The workshops are structured around memory-mapping, story-telling and turning autobiography into fiction. Performance poetry is very oriented towards the individual 'voice' – taking autobiography and creating drama out of it, using the facts and details of your life to create an emotional truth. It's an oral tradition where 'I' becomes the persona of a storyteller, relating experiences and observations to an equal audience.

We concentrate on childhood memories, hopes, fears, dreams and emotional responses, including a lot of humour and positivism in the writing. Paradoxically, this allows the women to explore some painful and difficult subjects that they had not talked about previously. These are not just about living with HIV, but also to do with childhood and upbringing, past and present relationships and living in a strange land where, for some, the threat of deportation looms nightmarishly. The poems about home, longing for Africa, for family, are complex for some because of the terrible circumstances in which they left, but for most, because if they were to return home, to see children or parents again, they would inevitably decline and die, because they would no longer have access to the medication that keeps their disease in check. Alongside this, I am really conscious of trying to make the sessions fun, of not putting any pressure on the writers to heave their hearts out onto the page, for the sake of my or anyone else's approval. These sessions are their time to meet. I feel really honoured that they have invited me into their circle and want to make sure that the sessions are not draining their energy.

I tell my poets that emotional truth is very important in their writing. That means that it touches people's hearts when they hear or read it. It feels real to them. But this does not mean that they have to tell facts about their own life. They can use their own under-standing of human nature to create fictional characters that seem to 'come off the page', 'are three-dimensional' or feelings that everyone shares, however different they are from you. This is the art of the writer.

We look at structure, using contrasts like past with present, humour with seriousness, happiness with sadness. I remind them each session that poets can change details, facts, places, names. We can write in a very abstract way so that there are no people in our poem, just emotions, colours, feelings, no 'I' or 'You'.

During the four sessions, it strikes me that these women are living with an illness that clouds over who they are and becomes a new and imposed identity. In my show, 'Chinese Whispers', I explore notions of identity; what makes us who we are – parents, birthplace, colour, sex, formative memories, name, nationality, language – none of which we tend to have any real choice over. As poets, we are able to resist, question or change the identity that has been given to us by the world. As performers, we are able to play with the paradox that we, ourselves, real people, are speaking our made-up works of fiction, often based on our own experiences, in the 'character' of ourselves.

When I ask the women if they would like to perform their work, I am thrilled to find that they do. I think that it's because the work is a) good and b) represents each writer in a way with which she feels comfortable. I know from my own experience that writing things down can be a way of exorcising painful memories from which one feels powerless to move on. We have done an exercise around this. However, I also feel that this particular set of workshops were to do with finding the poetic 'voice', rather than expressly using writing as a therapeutic tool. I hope that the sessions have been nurturing and possibly even healing, but the way they have been presented and structured is as creative writing masterclasses. I think that performance poetry is uniquely able to offer this possibility because it is a truly democratic art form. Anyone with a voice and something to say, can, if they are willing to put the work in, engage an audience with their story. Their voice may be cracked, their story might be difficult, but if they put their hearts, minds and imaginations into communicating it to their peers, they will capture the hearts, minds and imagination of an audience.

The next two workshops are about taking the writing into performance. We discuss what performance poetry is – for me, it's simply a poem or piece of writing that communicates 'live' to an audience. We discuss poems that don't work as performances as well as think-ing about poems that do. Poems that do might include some of the following:

- rhythm, rhyme and patterns – structures that enable the audience to 'work' during the piece, devices that engage the brain and ask the listener to participate in an active way
- narrative – again, a story helps to engage the audience actively – the piece is then a journey which happens in the present time
- imagery – paints a picture in the mind of the listener
- musicality – makes the listening experience pleasurable

- comedy – entertaining
- emotion – appealing and dramatic, draws the listener in
- politics/current affairs – a debate is set up.

The Poet as Performer becomes a persona during the performance – therefore, we think about non-verbal language and communication, physical appearance, body language, costume and staging. The women decide that they want to perform as a group. Together, we structure a series of individual pieces into a group poem around the theme of 'Life'. Some pieces are set in the past, others the present. Some are abstract and lyrical, others comic monologues with elements of audience participation. Some are introspective and personal, others political. The group chooses a name – 'African Ladies of London'.

Lucinda and her team work hard to ensure that the group are as comfortable as possible on the day, co-ordinating taxis, arrival times, sound checks and refreshments. The group arrive at the Riverside Studios, in Hammersmith in the afternoon and we spend some hours rehearsing in the space. It is important the women feel as relaxed and confident as possible. They get a basic lesson in microphone technique – for most of them, it will be their first time speaking into one and I make sure that they get the chance to hear how their voice sounds when speaking very close compared with further away. We work with the technical staff to set the lights, getting them acclimatised to the strange feeling of smiling and speaking into a sea of dazzling darkness. I tell them that we can turn the house-lights up so that they can make out the faces of the watching crowd, but that they should try and sense the audience – feel whether they are listening and listen to them smiling. I ask them to read their pieces again and again, so that they know them by heart. I encourage them to talk to individual members of the audience, smile at them, use gestures, eye-contact. I tell them that no matter how prepared we are, something will go not according to plan – they must try to go with it, enjoy it – if they are happy, then the audience will be happy.

One woman has second thoughts – not to do with disclosure, but because she is suddenly filled with a terrible sense of fear of failure. Interestingly, she comes across as the most confident member of the group. It is often the case that assertive and in control people are the ones intimidated by the idea of facing an audience, where shy and diffident people can be relatively free on stage. The group rally round with words of comfort and support. Somehow, they persuade her to take part. There is a sense from all of us that this performance symbolises the journey that we have gone on during our creative writing workshops. With any first-time performance poet, it's a huge act of ownership and empowerment to stand up and 'represent' – with this group in particular, the freedom and courage that they show by performing their work is exhilarating. And the fact that their piece is celebratory is a celebration of their personal and political choices.

Lucinda arranges a backstage area where we can relax and get into costume. Some of the Ladies buy wine and we sit, eating houmus and sipping Merlot from plastic cups in a buzz of pre-show adrenaline. Suzy can't make it, but she has sent lots of love. Katherine arrives on her bike! At last, the moment has arrived – the house lights dim, the audience settles down. I introduce the group 'African Ladies of London'– they take the stage, looking fabulous in colourful costumes. They are confident, charismatic, witty and moving. They get a huge round of applause. Afterwards, they are congratulated by many members of the audience. I am very proud.

After Rosetta Live! I miss working with the group. I apply to BBC Radio 4 to write a radio drama in conjunction with a community group, namely, African Ladies of London.

The play is commissioned as part of a programme called 'Stages of Sound'. It enables me to carry on working with the group through the rest of the year. 'The Healing Pool', written in conjunction with some of the African Ladies of London, was broadcast on Radio 4 and London Live in May 2005.

Suzy Croft is a senior social worker at St John's Palliative Care Centre and Research Fellow at the Centre for Citizen Participation at Brunel University. She is a trustee of two leading UK palliative care organisations and she is a member of the editorial collective of *Critical Social Policy*.

Francesca Beard is a London-based writer and performer on the international spoken-word circuit. She is currently touring her one-woman show, 'Chinese Whispers' and developing a new work for multiple voices, produced by Apples and Snakes with support from the Arts Council, England. She has worked extensively as a creative workshop facilitator both in Britain and abroad. To find out more about Francesca and her work, visit her website at www.francescabeard.com.

PART 3: ADVANCING INVOLVEMENT

Is There Anything Funny About Pain?

Pain. Payout.
Pain in the breadbasket not just in France
Now at your local village store!
Gut wrenching
Not in the neck
Not in the arse.
Pain. Payout.

Now just breathe...
In. Out. In. Out.
Piss off! I've been doing it since birth.
Don't need no lessons now.
Pain lessening is what I need.

Coax. Make friends.
Welcome it as part of life
Of being alive
Payout pain.
Savour its sweetness
Careful with its sharp edges
Sink into its lushness but
Look out for haystack needles.
Welcome the clean smell
Just slightly spicy
A gamey edge.

'Pay In'
I know some people pay good money,
But I thought it was free.
Oh no, anything but free.
Safely contained
Uniquely experienced.
But what about the leaks?
(Oh yes, take them off the hob, will you dear?)
The grimaces in loving faces

The sleepless beige around dark eyes
The sharp intakes of breath
The tears
The forced smiles
Anyone, even me, can see that's pain.
Yes but only theirs.
They must breathe too
And one day they will.

Tout le pain a disparu
Crumbs only.
Where does it lurk, struggling with skeins of pharmacy-driven mayhem?
Playful.
Popping a pinch here, a flick there.
Reaching out to hug me
Like a bear who's rolled in pine needles
Kept at bay with a flimsy stick.
Smiling.
Teasing.
You know you like it.
Everyone deserves a bit of kinkiness.
I even have a soft French name:
Douleur.
Clouseau for American money.
Pay now and keep pain.
Keep paying till you reach the get out clause.
Oh yes.
Can I stop breathing now?

Paul Laking
December 2005

CHAPTER 11

Becoming involved in research: a service user research advisory group

Phil Cotterell, Paula Clarke,[1] Di Cowdrey, John Kapp, Mandy Paine and Rick Wynn

It was towards the end of 2002 when we came together, a group of service users who had differing life-limiting conditions and a researcher interested in palliative care issues. Some of the service users had a considerable lack of confidence, one or two had been through harrowing ordeals, but they shared a wide range of experience and knowledge. A common link between us all was a motivation to collectively undertake research with the aim of gaining accounts from people about their lives with life-limiting conditions, the services they needed, and their experience of relationships since diagnosis.

In this chapter we discuss our own experiences of becoming involved in this palliative care research project. This collaboration of service users and researcher involved us all working together as a team on the project. Members of the Service User Research Advisory Group (SURAG) were not the subjects of the research, nor were they interviewed as participants; rather they were involved to provide their perspective and their knowledge based on experience, on a wide range of research issues. They were members of the research team and assisted the research from the beginning of the project. The group was active at all stages including:

- designing the project and deciding what questions to ask
- assisting with how research information was collected
- making sense of the information (data analysis)
- teaching and writing about what we have done.

It was a novel idea as the involvement of service users in research was unusual within palliative care when this project began.

In writing this chapter together we have drawn on written extracts and audio-taped discussions about the project and the research. Phil has pulled the information together and written it down but the content originated from us all in SURAG and we have all been involved in editing this chapter. Comments from Phil were those written as the

---

[1] Paula Clarke's contribution to this writing is included as a result of her wishes prior to her death and of her partner's recent agreement.

research proceeded in his 'critical reflections' log and in other writings. Direct contributions are included in this chapter and attributed to the specific person concerned.

Coming together to work together

The research began as an idea of Phil's when he was working as a community nurse at a hospice (similar to what is known as a 'Macmillan Nurse'). He worked in a team based at a hospice but would visit people in their own homes to offer advice on symptoms they were experiencing and fulfil a supportive role. The emphasis of the hospice was on people with cancer and motor neurone disease. Sometimes this work with these people and their families would span several months and consequently Phil got to know some people very well indeed. Over time Phil became very aware that people with other conditions such as chronic lung conditions or those who were HIV+, had palliative care needs and that locally ways of addressing these needs were underdeveloped. He was also aware that many patients wanted a greater say in the way the hospice was run and in what services it, and other providers of care and support, offered.

These two areas became the focus of the research in the beginning. However, he also wanted to ensure that the research would be of use to people who might need palliative care. He wanted to ensure that the research was in tune with what service users wanted or thought could be useful. He decided to ask people themselves what they thought.

Local service users were asked about the initial research ideas and questions and it was Di, who later became active in the research as a member of SURAG, who suggested bringing together local service user groups. Meeting Di was pivotal for Phil as he explained:

> I met someone who was determined to promote service users' views in order to maximise services available to people, and she was also passionate about helping with the research and trying to improve things for people who have palliative care needs. Meeting Di early on when I was thinking about the research and formulating questions helped me to clarify research questions and to think about how the research might work with service users working alongside me on the project.

This meeting to discuss the initial research idea and questions aimed to establish if these service user representatives agreed that the research questions were worth pursuing or whether there were other key concerns to focus on. They did agree with the overall research aim and questions and SURAG was formed.

Local people were invited by letter to join SURAG, or to be interviewed for the research. With the letter was a newsletter giving more in-depth information. More than 300 letters and newsletters were circulated to local service user and support groups, religious groups, hospital consultants, specialist nurses, community district nurses, and general practitioners, as well as to social service and mental health organisations and individuals. The intention was to tell as wide a range of people as possible about the research, as well as prompting them to discuss it with service users.

The first service users interested in the research chose whether to join SURAG *or* be interviewed as a research participant. Once eight people had been recruited to SURAG, the rest were asked to take part in interviews or small group discussions. SURAG first met in November 2002 and the first interviews began in January 2003. The research was beginning ...

Our first meeting

Phil explained the role of SURAG to its eight members, and acknowledged that it would develop over time under the members' influence. Four of the members attended the same hospice day centre and so knew each other a little; the other four members, plus Phil, knew no one in the group.

Looking back it is clear that there was a lack of understanding about what people were getting involved in. One member, Paula, had Chronic Obstructive Pulmonary Disease (COPD). She and some others had not fully realised that they were not going to be interviewed but that their role was quite different. Paula explained that, because she was so nervous before the first meeting, she had not read properly the information she had been given, such as the draft 'Terms of Reference' document. She was terrified about the meeting because she had lost confidence as a result of a recent hospital experience when she had been extremely unwell. She had nearly died and was in intensive care for three months. Previously she had been very confident, but was unsure now how she would react to people and respond to being in a group again and whether she would be listened to. Paula was also concerned that her mind wasn't as sharp as it used to be, and that she might not be able to think clearly. 'I'd had the rug pulled out from under me' she said.

She also worried about the location. Would it be on one level? Could she take oxygen and nasal cannula in with her? She recalled certain anxieties about the meeting and said, 'I didn't want to make a fool of myself'. Paula felt that there could have been more planning and explanation about the first meeting, and more thought given to the members' concerns and requirements:

> I was frightened about taking my coat off (in the meeting), so didn't. I wasn't sure if I'd be able to go and get it at the end of the meeting. Would it be upstairs?

On reflection it is clear that preparation could have been a lot better. Phil didn't fully appreciate the members' experiences of ill health and its affect on them, even though he had a lot of experience in working with people with advanced life-limiting conditions. However Paula did recall that the first meeting was comforting:

> When everybody started introducing themselves I thought maybe they are as nervous as I am, 'lets just go with this'. Once I realised it was perfectly normal people, not a big professional body, it wasn't a scary place to be. I relaxed and I thoroughly enjoyed it and I've fed off it ever since, I look forward to going enormously. Once I realised no physical demands were going to be made of me, there was nothing I was going to have to say that I couldn't think of an answer to, if I didn't have an answer I didn't have to say anything it didn't matter, it was OK.

Paula recalled that she knew the meeting was about research but that she was not sure what was expected of her. Once in the group she knew she wasn't going to be a research participant, although it took a while to fully realise this. She also said that she felt pleased there were people with conditions other than COPD, as you don't always want to see others with the same condition and she had worried about this. It's about choosing how much to see and learn about your own condition. However, in reality, it was rewarding to see someone like Mandy who had been through so much and was coping and getting on with life. She said it inspired her, although this was tinged with some fear, which was about seeing the future for herself. Paula reflected, however, that she became inspired and positive about the future rather than negative. She also felt that mixing with people who have cancer was not an issue at all, as she had experience of cancer in her own family.

John had been a carer until his partner's death, and is also a member of a Cancer Network Patients Forum Group. Reflecting on the first SURAG meeting he said:

> I was looking forward to the first meeting, I felt quite privileged to be asked to join. If I hadn't nursed Janet through her terminal illness and seen her deterioration, her emaciation and pain and so on, I think I might have found it difficult to cope with, some of the group members who have got breathing apparatus and are clearly in pain some of the time. It is hard sometimes because of the mirror effect, but there for the grace of God go you.

Rick had lung cancer, and knew some of the people who went to the group from the hospice day centre that he attended. He described himself as an outgoing sort of person and looked forward to the first meeting. Rick was surprised by some of the other members' disabilities, such as difficulty with walking and difficulty with breathing. He recalled Mandy using oxygen from a cylinder. He was also surprised that these people were also involved in other things. He thought they were very brave. Rick said that he didn't expect to see people who were obviously so ill saying, 'mine's not obvious but theirs is'. He was surprised that they were there at all, and said:

> I felt proud of them, that they were there.

This was not a patronising comment at all, but rather conveyed a genuine sense of respect and, in a way, gratitude. Gratitude that people with serious conditions would get involved in trying to improve things for others. As Paula had mentioned, Rick felt that more explanation at the outset of what was wrong with people, and their role in the group, would have been helpful. He didn't know what COPD meant and thought it was good that it wasn't all people with cancer, that there was a cross-section of conditions. Rick felt that it was a good idea to have this cross-section and to be focusing on palliative care needs for various conditions and not purely cancer.

Mandy has COPD and remembers explaining about her COPD condition at the start of the first meeting. She said that people didn't understand what it was and that she didn't understand other illnesses, so this early discussion gave us increased understanding. She felt that 'at the end of the day we were all pretty similar'. In advance of the meeting she recalled:

> I was quite nervous. I wondered what it was all about. I thought I've got nothing to lose. I suddenly felt like a new person ... I suppose I didn't feel ... I felt nervous the first meeting but when I got there I didn't feel like a square peg in a round hole.

Mandy was also anxious about whether she was going to cope with meeting people she didn't know:

> I hadn't met new people for a long time. I also felt excited, suddenly I didn't feel that I would be alone because there might be somebody there who's got the same as me and I wouldn't be alone any more, which has happened.

Mandy also recalled being very interested in the research and its aims:

I like to investigate things and understand how things work or how things evolve, that bit's interesting, that perhaps something would be out there. The fact that I'm now getting involved with it, it doesn't feel negative any more. It's quite daunting when you first come in though with a room of people you've never met before.

At the time of the first meeting Di was the Vice-Chair of West Sussex Disability Network and also had COPD. She also reflected on the first meeting of SURAG:

At the first meeting of the user advisory group it felt good when I realised that Phil was going out and researching with other people not on the members of the group. It was explained clearly at that meeting that this was the case and that accounts from these participants would be brought back to the group anonymously.

She also commented on meeting with people who had different conditions from herself in the group:

People were so positive. Someone with a brain tumour was so positive, to me that was a lot worse than me suffering a lung disorder, the tumour on the brain; it could be stopping activity, stopping her thinking but she was so positive. It had an effect on me. It came to me that people who have life-threatening diseases are looking at the world with a much more positive view than anybody else seems to. They've got all these problems, they know that one day their life is going to end, perhaps a bit nastily, and yet they are so positive to help other people. I saw members grow in confidence in the group. Everyone has brought a different angle into the group. Your own problem seems to take a back seat in a way. It's always there for you but when you come you are interested in what they have to say and looking at it from their point of view.

Di also recalls some of her initial concerns about joining the group:

I was a little bit worried coming to the first meeting but there was such a nice lot of people there. I really looked forward to the next meeting. If people weren't talking much you could tell that they were following what was being said and were interested.

Prior to the first meeting a draft 'Terms of Reference' document was circulated and an agenda explaining that this and the role of the advisory group would be discussed and agreed at the meeting. Also Phil had spoken individually with everyone about the research and SURAG's proposed role in the research. This was deliberately left somewhat vague in order that the group would have scope to alter this and shape it for themselves. Phil's initial reaction to the first meeting was very different from some of the service user members discussed above:

YES ... It went very well. Everyone got on well together from the outset. We started by introducing ourselves ... The time went very quickly for me. We stopped for refreshments halfway through and there was good discussion between everyone and a friendly atmosphere. I felt very comfortable with everyone and from my perspective it felt good to all be together. I hope everyone else felt similarly. Good points were raised about the key purpose of the research, time-scale and expected outcomes. There was a general consensus that people need to hear how it is for people living with many different conditions and that services are often inadequate. The research needs to lead to change, which means the findings will have to be presented to the right people.

Phil was surprised when he heard later about members' anxieties about the meeting, as described above. He had felt that everyone was prepared and his anxieties had been different:

> I got a buzz from this meeting. Everyone was up for it and it all seemed to flow well. My anxiety was around how people would get on together and find the group but this was relieved very soon as people seemed at ease with each other and the idea of the group. Everyone participated; some more than others, which I suppose, is to be expected. There appeared to be a collective move to get things rolling.

Doing this for me, doing this for you

Why would people with so many pressing issues themselves become involved in a project such as this? There are a number of reasons why people agreed to take part, and have continued to give their time and energy. Mandy describes being curious, but also she saw it as a form of escape from her own situation. When she joined the research group she felt more in touch with herself:

> What motivated me ... curiosity I suppose. It was an escape from it all, going to something away from the situation you were in ... being a person, when I'm at the meeting, I'm me. I'm not my son's mother or my husband's wife or my parent's child, I'm me. When you're working, you're you, aren't you. When we come to the meetings we ... we're getting involved, we're part of the group, part of a unit really, you become an individual, become a person, and also, where the illness was a real negative, a real downer, being involved has stopped that being a real downer. All right, it's within you, it's not fun ... but at least I know I'm going to leave my mark, so this was a way of leaving my mark. From the first meeting I thought I could actually make a difference, if I get involved in this, part of my being involved will make a difference for somebody else. It was something that was missing that I badly needed. When I was told what I'd got it would have been nice to have been handed something or understood a bit more about it, perhaps this will help, it will also help doctors and nurses etc.

From the outset Mandy had an idea, not only about leaving her own mark so that others would remember her, but also that lessons would be learnt from her own experience and the experiences of the research participants. She has spoken in terms of striving to make a smoother path on which others with similar conditions could travel. Involvement was clearly linked to action for change then. She has been clear that this difference or action for others is for the future, for people who will come after she has died. Mandy further remarks:

> We were all in the same boat and you can support each other if you're having a bad day. It was a bit scary to start with until they explained what it was and you under-stood it. I used to get anxious before the first couple of meetings and self conscious

of bringing oxygen cylinders with me. Worried that you might look stupid in front of everybody if you didn't understand something, but that didn't happen. We all explained everything. There was a lot of paperwork ... reading it all, but I have got the hang of it now. It was a problem in case I forgot anything that I had written down. The first meeting there was a lot of paper to take in, the terms of reference. I hoped I wouldn't break any rules. Not talking about it with family was a concern, confidentiality.

Mandy also felt that there was a difference between the members of the group who had cancer and others with different conditions:

The first meeting did feel a bit them and us. Our side and their side (of the room).

Di outlined another perspective about involvement in SURAG:

What's amazed me, although we all have our different illnesses, the things that are lacking in services etc. are basically the same no matter what the condition. The only difference that comes through in the research is that there is more support for cancer patients than there has been for any other condition. The cancer patients interviewed have said what wonderful support and those with other life-threatening conditions say the support is not there. That has definitely come through in the research. There is not the expertise coming round to see them at home. You have the GP, but sometimes you want to talk things over, not just about your illness, but also about your family. It's been a very interesting time of my life. Since doing this work I realise that patients that have gone home still suffer in some shape or form and not seen.

Membership of the group has had a positive effect on Paula:

I feel valuable again. It makes me feel like I can do something again. I know what I'm not able to do any more so, if I'm any use at all, I'm pleased. The interviews and presentation of them in the summaries are a good idea. They make you think a bit more about them, you can feed off them and it promotes discussion. It links into your own experience and you can agree or think, I don't see it that way.

Paula also has hopes for the outcomes of the research:

A lot of people interviewed don't have the strong family I do. The research might draw that point out – how important social support is. It must be mind-blowing if you don't have that facility. You need somebody who is sympathetic, will listen and not treat you as a patient all the time. Support and support groups is a most important part of living with a life-limiting condition. We have seen what is important to interviewees and where there are gaps in services. This will all become clear when the research ends.

Being in the group has had a positive effect on its members. This raised awareness of the experiences of others can potentially lead to wider effects. Group members have continued to strive for positive changes to come from the research, with some taking positive steps to establish and develop a support/campaigning group. Although there have been supportive aspects to membership of SURAG, it has not been a support group. This was clear in the group's 'Terms of Reference' document. It was very much a working group. It has also contributed to the personal development of SURAG members and Phil, as he has described:

> Service users benefited by way of their own personal development, their changed sense of themselves in comparison to others, in a sort of sense of solidarity and belonging, and in the support found within SURAG plus in other ways. I benefited by meeting all the SURAG members, learning from them and with them, developing friendships, and in gaining fuller and different perspectives about living with the conditions they and participants live with. The research benefited throughout but particularly at the analysis and theme generation phase when the direction of the research and its findings really did shift.

Being involved in the team changed people's perspectives and understanding.

My experience, becomes our experience, becomes our knowledge

Di identified how the group members' own experiences can merge with the experiences of people taking part in the research. Paula commented on how the group gained from reading the research interviews:

> When we were reading these interviews we said 'yes I can empathise with this because of my experience'. Looking at the questions we have been asking and for us looking at them and saying, 'yes that's true, yes I've suffered that'. A lot of familiar things are seen in the interview accounts. It has made me angry at times thinking 'why hasn't this happened to them'.

Di adds more about joint experiences:

> It's been a full working research group. Sometimes we have been distracted and Phil has let that happen. Although we haven't always finished as much work as planned in the meeting because of having the time to talk about our own experiences has helped everybody.

Although talking about participants' experiences and group members' experiences can help, there can also be some difficulties. Di went on:

> Sometimes if you see something brought up from a participant you think 'Yeah, yeah I can go with that' but you've never spoken about it before, you never talk about it and I think that is why it has helped. Even if you don't speak out at the meeting, it's gone into your head and you can work it out and then you can tell someone, GP or family member, if you want to. I think you have to be careful with yourself that you don't take on other people's problems and make them yours if they are not there. Sometimes I think this hasn't happened to me thank God. If you are that type of person, it could give you a symptom that is not really there. If it gets to you too much, you are not any good for the group, but this group seems to be quite strong.

The research as it unfolded and progressed became a developmental process in which we were all involved. It was not only the research that developed, but also us as individuals, and as a group of people with a common aim. Our understanding has developed. Understanding about our own conditions, understanding about living with the conditions in the research, understanding about working together as very different people but people with common aims, hopes and ambitions. Collectively we have been better able to see the situation of living with a life-limiting condition. As a result, we have identified opportunities for improvements that are highlighted as recommendations of the research.

Phil has noted how SURAG members' experiences combined with the research participants' experiences have developed into their own form of knowledge:

> [SURAG] members illustrated belief in what they knew, particularly when faced with data from participants that echoed their own experiences; here they also showed intuitive understanding about a whole range of issues and experiences participants spoke of. There was also a clear awareness, for some group members, about their own developing skills; and lastly there was a raised realisation about their own and others' situations.

It does upset you

Two main things have had the potential to upset members of the group. One is the ill health and death of fellow group members and the other is what the interviewees have said. Di sums this up:

> When we have lost people (SURAG members) it really upset me. It's bound to affect us. It does bring it up that one day it will be you.

Others have been more philosophical. Paula said, 'I was expecting one or two people not to be there all the time' and John said, 'I think it is a natural thing that has to happen'.

For Mandy the ill health and death of fellow SURAG members raised several different issues:

> I have through the group really made some lovely friends. When [name] died it really did hit us badly. It's also hard about [name] as he has done so much for us. We have felt the pain with him ... you know your own pain and you're thinking that's what it's like for him. Desperately wanting to help him.

In this group these issues have had to be dealt with, as the people involved are very ill. Reflecting on this led Mandy to say:

> How much of the group is helping us have an extension of our life? How much is it giving us something to fight for? I know it is me. There are days when I feel 'I really don't want to carry on' and then I think 'come on pull yourself together, you've got this to do ...' and it makes you think 'come on'. At the same time sometimes you do want to give up but then you do feel if you do that you'll be letting people down (other group members).

Despite this emotional aspect of involvement, or because of it, Mandy never considered giving up the group. She did wonder what effect these deaths had on other group members though. Perhaps group members who were particularly close to someone that died might feel like ceasing their involvement. This has recently proved not to be the case though following Paula's death. This distressed us all and we all attended her funeral and keep her very much in mind when we meet. This is especially so as the research is coming to its conclusion.

The research data from participants has also been challenging at times. Over the course of the research the group has seen the anonymised transcripts of what people said in the interviews and group discussions, and these have sometimes contained troubling accounts from participants. Mandy describes her thoughts on this:

> Sometimes you feel you want to go and give them a ring and say 'look you're not on your own' which can't happen because of confidentiality, others you feel like saying don't just lay back and be ill, and there's others you're thinking 'hey sit down, have a rest, let others take over'.

Mandy goes on to speak about one particular participant that left a lasting impression on her:

> We felt bitterly for him that he was on his own.

And another participant who raised angry feelings in her:

> It was the way the system was treating her. Having been there myself I knew exactly where she was coming from. I think with this research it's made us all quite ecstatic towards people. Quite a few people we have really felt for, we have wanted to be there for them and we have felt angry about the services, how they have treated them. There was the lady who had different carers everyday and she had to explain each time how it was done...

SURAG members were not directly involved in data collection and Mandy went on to consider the one-sided perspective this may offer:

> We haven't met the person, we haven't been able to read them as well as read what they are saying. It does bring up quite strong feelings. Sometimes you get a feeling of really wanting to help them, and that sort of feeling of helplessness. But also a mixed feeling at the same time of understanding where they are coming from. You suddenly want to write a letter to their social worker and have a go at them. That's when we ring each other (group members).

Di felt similarly:

> A lot of familiar things are seen in the interview accounts. It has made me angry at times thinking why hasn't this happened to them.

This impact was also experienced by Paula:

> Some accounts from interviewees are pretty hard hitting. It isn't necessarily what I would feel but it's desperately sad for them. I don't recall ever not being able to say I can understand them feeling that way. I can understand what they are saying.

Being upset to some degree has been a part of this project for SURAG members, either about members of SURAG itself or about research participants whose accounts we have read in interview transcripts. SURAG members expressed the impact of these things on themselves and this was dealt with as a group either in or outside the group. Friendships developed amongst group members and much informal support was offered between group meetings. This was not led by Phil but developed as an important aspect of the research. Within group meetings support was offered by everyone when appropriate. As previously mentioned, support was not the overriding purpose of the group but was needed due to the nature of the research. SURAG members did not attend the meetings to gain personal support, but this was offered as part of a caring group as issues arose. There was a general acceptance that different things would affect different people in different ways. Emotion, and the expression of it, was seen as a part of living with the conditions SURAG members and research participants had.

Phil had anxieties about the SURAG members at times, and there was a gradual shift from a fairly paternalistic position to a more equal and democratic position. Early on in the 'life' of the group he wrote:

> In the group today it was strikingly evident that people are very ill. Am I expecting too much?

A little later, in considering two members going to present with him at a conference in London about service users getting involved in research, he added:

> There is a big personal cost involved. Both are going in with their eyes opened though. Mandy is particularly 'up' for the conference and praising of SURAG and me for giving her the opportunity to 'come out of herself' and focus on 'things out there rather than just be negative and inward looking.' This is how she was, she says, before SURAG. I found it very moving talking to her on the phone today. I am concerned as to what I have started in a way and then I think perhaps I'm being a bit paternal and 'nursey'. It seems that the process people are embarked upon is giving a great deal of personal meaning and purpose.

There was also a time when he felt some merging between professional and personal roles:

> I have been thinking about my relationships with members of SURAG. I am getting close and friendly with members and it feels like my professional role/identity is being challenged. This is not a negative thing I guess but a consequence of the service user involvement approach I am taking in this project.

It would be incorrect though to think that being upset or having concerns have been the main features of this project, but this is discussed here to honestly illustrate the various issues faced in such a project.

What have we done?

The SURAG members and Phil have worked on many different things connected to the research. At the beginning, group members helped to reshape the interview questions and advised on the way interviews were conducted. They also contributed to data interpretation and the general monitoring and progress of the research. The interpretation of research data was in fact a very complex and prolonged phase of the project that highlighted the commitment of members to the project. This phase of interpreting the data or making sense of the data, and then agreeing on research findings took nine months.

Some group members have also been involved in a range of teaching opportunities about the research and how we were doing it. This has been locally for professionals and service user groups, but also at national conferences.

As a result of people's involvement in the group and their work on this research, opportunities have also arisen for members to teach in other settings as well, and to get involved in other initiatives separate from this research. Some SURAG members are clear that involvement in this research group has increased their confidence greatly. An idea of the range of things that SURAG members have contributed to is given here:

▥ help with the phrasing of interview questions
▥ giving insights based on their own experiences, about participants responses
▥ reflections on whether we were gaining the information we had hoped for
▥ raising important points about the research data as we reviewed it
▥ commenting and advising on the researchers' style and level of sensitivity to participants
▥ great involvement in making sense of all the data (data analysis)
▥ involvement with teaching about the research and the process.

As the research proceeded, some members wanted to become more involved and wanted to see participants when they were interviewed. To this end, honorary contracts were obtained from the local NHS trust but this unfortunately was only organised towards the end of the data collection process, and there were not the opportunities for this level of involvement. On one day when Phil was to be accompanied to interview a participant, the SURAG member due to come was unfortunately too unwell. A regret of Phil's is not enabling wider involvement in the research at an earlier stage of the project.

Nevertheless, involvement in the project has enthused group members. It has enabled members to see things differently, and it has motivated members to campaign for improvements. Di illustrated this point when she was considering what it is she takes from the experience of being involved in the research:

> Looking at life in a different way, knowing you are not on your own, wanting to go and speak to the Government to get more money (for palliative care), educate all that are involved in the caring and nursing of people with life-threatening conditions. Working together has been fantastic and has proven that service users can work with any professional people.

In Di's view, professionals working with service users need to care about what they are doing and for the service users involved. A good relationship with the professionals is the most important factor in making involvement successful for service users. Phil agrees and adds that one of the most valuable contributions from service users involved in research is their commitment and hope, particularly in palliative care research. Researchers need to understand service users in this area, be commited themselves to collaborative working, and hope for change or action as a result of their project.

Conclusion

SURAG members have learned a lot from their involvement in the research project and have hopes for its impact. John highlights this:

> I think one of the purposes of the research and the group is our own personal development. I feel that my own development has taken notches further forward by interaction with this group. What I would hope for from this group … its about a benefit for society, an effect on the outside world … if we can reach to other depths that are normally skated over, we want to make people who read this report suddenly open their eyes and say 'I've never seen that in print before, I've never thought of that before'. That is the sort of thing I would like to come out of this research.

Rick also clearly sees the need for the research to lead to positive action for others:

> We are gathering this information, not just to record it, but to pass it on to a department that can do exactly what that person is in need of. As a group we need to be thinking of passing on information about the gaps that we are finding.

There has always been a real sense from all group members of wanting to do this for other people with similar conditions. Mandy highlights this point:

> It will make a difference, it is gaining an insight into what we live with, like a fly on the wall. Hopefully it will give people courage to speak up later (when they read the report). It might open a gate to better communication between professionals and service users and it might open a gate to improving services. It might prompt people in these areas.

She also reflects on the conclusion of the project:

> Although we are coming to the end of the research I want to start the next volume. We've put the foundations down and now we need to start building up. The next step is getting the research out there and getting people to read it and to listen to us. We are getting people to listen to us already (i.e. conferences and talks).

The research findings include six main themes, briefly described below.

1 Diagnosis. All participants described the traumatic period around receiving their diagnosis. It shocked them and some struggled with whom to tell about their condition, how much information to give and a range of other issues.
2 Emotions. They described strong emotions including fear, grief, anger and frustration. Some had thoughts of dying and fears about losing independence, lacking control and frustrations about the care and support they would receive. Some were angry about the unrelenting, and all too visible, progression of their condition. Many recounted losses and a deep sorrowfulness. For many these feelings were not purely in response to physical changes, but were also in response to social changes, such as the change in relationships with some friends and family members.
3 Relationships. We heard of challenges to relationships. Participants told us how, as restrictions were enforced upon them by their condition, some friends dropped away.

Some responses from friends were extreme and unexpected, and some participants felt they were being seen for their condition and their impairments rather than for themselves. These changes in relationships led to a degree of social withdrawal for many.

4   Services. Participants talked about a wide range of services including community, hospital, hospice and social care, and the staff delivering them. They told us about what they received and what they felt they needed. There were many examples of good practice from staff, with participants valuing respectful and helpful staff. There were examples of effective and beneficial services. Unfortunately, there were many more examples of services and staff that were below standard.

5   Difference/individuality. Participants felt that they were seen and treated as different following diagnosis of their condition whilst they strived to maintain their own individuality. Many participants needed to accept care and support from health and/or social care staff but they still tried to be self-governing and to retain their self-esteem.

6   Being independent or dependent. The last theme of independent/dependent conveys participants' efforts to maintain independence despite increasing levels of dependence on others and on services. Participants told of their attempts to counter paternalistic carers and to convey the specifics of their condition and needs. We saw a tension here with participants needing to accept care and support, but also needing to have control, choice and to retain decision-making powers. Having control and choice, despite having physical restrictions, was seen to offer independence.

A report of the research carries recommendations for health and social care staff. The findings reflect the value of having service users involved in the research, particularly at the stage of analysing the data analysis.

In summary, we have shown that the service users who were involved in this research as members of the advisory group, brought much passion, commitment and insight to the project. In the area of palliative care it is easy to be paternalistic about involving service users in research and other areas. Undoubtedly, ensuring people are safe and are not taken advantage of because of their goodwill, is essential, especially when they are very ill. However, this does not mean that the option or choice to be involved should be taken from people. Clearly service users involved in this project have not only helped and added to the research, but have also gained much personally and collectively.

Phil acknowledges the work involved in developing such a group and in achieving more equal relationships as opposed to maintaining a traditional professional/patient type role. He has needed to challenge some of his own attitudes and doubts. The whole group has been instrumental in developing relationships whereby all can contribute, be heard, valued, and empowered to develop and to be involved as much as they want to be or are able to be. To empathise with participants but to keep the purpose of the project in mind has also needed work over our time together.

We acknowledge that the ending of the project and the group brings its own difficulties. It has been a significant part of our lives and, as well as producing research findings, the group has had a life of its own in which all of us have received much support, guidance, and friendship. A new challenge on the horizon is to address all our needs at the conclusion of the project. The project has taken up a great deal of time and energy for all involved and has come to symbolise different things for different people. Involvement is continuing in a different form for some SURAG members who are developing a support/mutual aid group for people with life-limiting conditions. This new initiative has evolved from the work undertaken in the research. We would also like to be involved in further collaborative research.

Acknowledgments

We would like to acknowledge the involvement and important contribution made by all previous members of the Service User Research Advisory Group who participated during the course of the project.

Phil Cotterell is a Research Fellow in Palliative Care at Worthing and Southlands Hospitals NHS Trust. He worked with the Service User Research Advisory Group (SURAG) to complete a research project that was known as the 'Influencing Palliative Care Project'. This group involved a researcher and service users with a range of long-term/life-limiting conditions working together over a three-year period to find out what people with progressive conditions like cancer, stroke, HIV+ and respiratory conditions identified as their needs and to find out more about these people's experiences of health and social care services and life with their particular condition.

The aim of SURAG was to ensure that the research remained in tune with service user concerns and needs, and to enable group members to influence the research at all stages of the research process. The group was active at all stages, from the design of the project through to telling people about our research findings. This joining together to carry out research is particularly unusual in palliative care. The group consisted of nine people in all over the time span of the project, with most group members dealing with the consequences of advanced conditions. Indeed four of the original members died over the course of the project.

Users as educators: how hospice patients can help in the training of health professionals

Emma Hall and Jennifer Todd

Introduction

Patients have been successfully involved in the education and training of doctors and other health professionals (HPs) for many years. However, until about 15 years ago, patient participation in education was largely passive. There are also ethical concerns around the need to balance the educational needs of health professionals with the rights of potentially vulnerable patients. The question of remuneration has also been raised, particularly if the patient has entered a formal training programme, and this is discussed in a recent literature review.[1]

The Department of Health (DoH) report 'The Expert Patient'[2] highlighted the need for patients with chronic disease to be seen as both 'partners' and 'experts' in their condition, rather than passive recipients of healthcare.

The acquisition and demonstration of excellent communication skills now forms an essential part of the training of HPs. The government has recognised the importance of HPs in *all* specialties attaining such skills in the DoH publications 'The NHS Knowledge and Skills Framework (NHS KSF)' in 2004, and 'Curriculum for the foundation years in postgraduate education and training' in 2005.[3]

The importance of sensitive communication of bad news, the need to listen to patients' and carers' concerns, discussion of therapeutic interventions, and properly informed consent have been emphasised particularly in cancer and palliative care,[4] although these are essential for all aspects of health and social care.

This chapter will focus mainly on the teaching of communication skills, although reference to other aspects of HP training will also be given.

The teachers will most often be referred to as 'patients', rather than 'users', because the term 'patient' is used in most of the literature. One study of patients accessing general practitioners and psychiatrists suggested that patients themselves prefer this term to 'user' or 'customer'.[5] It should be noted that carers have been involved in teaching, and this is also discussed.

Communication skills teaching – why is it important?

Good communication skills are essential for HPs, in order to develop a trusting therapeutic relationship with their patients. There is a suggestion from research, that these skills are not always instinctive, and that formal teaching using a variety of methods is often very beneficial.

Evidence from a recent systematic review suggests that oncology (cancer) doctors and nurses who receive formal communication skills training, tend to ask more open questions and express themselves more empathically, than those who do not receive such training. However, it should be noted that the authors identified only 3 eligible trials out of 2824 references, and were unable to comment on long-term efficacy of the training.[6]

The majority of communication skills training in cancer care has focused on qualified doctors and nurses, and has usually involved the use of role-play and actors. There has been concern that many patients who have cancer or other serious diseases, may be too ill to participate in this type of training. However, a number of recent initiatives working with hospice patients have challenged this view. The valuable contribution to training that they can make has been highlighted, not just for undergraduates but also for qualified HPs.

Medical and nursing schools have started to include formal teaching on communication skills in their curricula, to emphasise the importance of introducing this subject as early in a career as possible.

What can palliative care professionals learn from other specialties?

A recent literature review identified 23 studies involving patients as teachers.[1] Communication skills was one of many aspects of healthcare covered, but others included:

- physical examination skills
- developmental disabilities in children
- dementia
- mental health
- HIV (Human immunodeficiency virus) disease.

In general practice and psychiatry, the learning of communication skills with patients as teachers is well established. In general practice, trainees are expected to submit a series of videoed consultations with patients, as part of their assessment process. The use of 'consumer examiners' in one study demonstrated the potential of patients to be as effective as doctors in assessing the communication skills of postgraduate trainees in general practice.[7]

In the field of psychiatry, it has become mandatory to include patients and carers in the teaching of postgraduate psychiatry trainees since 2005. Fadden *et al*[8] discuss several aspects of psychiatry training, in which patients may become involved as teachers:

- curriculum planning
- provision of feedback after clinical encounters
- qualitative comments on assignments
- involvement in recruitment and selection panels.

What are the potential advantages and disadvantages for patients of being involved in HP education?

There is evidence from qualitative studies that patients perceive a number of benefits from involvement in education of HPs. In a study of undergraduate medical student training in general practice, these included: a feeling of empowerment from being experts in their condition, altruism ('I'm giving something back'), positive feedback from students that feelings of distress were 'normal', and increased understanding of the doctor's role.[9]

Similar themes were identified in a qualitative study, which asked a user focus group for views on patients teaching pre-registration nursing students: for example one person said, '... it gives me confidence to stand up in front of trainee nurses', while another commented, 'I think the thing I enjoy, is that you can actually tell them the little things that would make your life easier'. In the same study, patients gave constructive feedback comments about timing and the need to ensure confidentiality issues; adjustments to future teaching sessions were made as a result.[10]

Perceived disadvantages for patients as teachers include: concerns about confidentiality, lack of remuneration, inconvenience, and exhaustion from repeated sessions.

What are the advantages and disadvantages to learners of being taught by patients?

Wykurz and Kelly summarise the advantages to learners as: deepened understanding, increased knowledge of services and chronic conditions, the opportunity to receive constructive feedback from patients, improved confidence, increased respect and empathy, and a positive influence on behaviour and attitude.[1]

Disadvantages to learners were not discussed in this review, but anecdotally the authors have noted concerns from learners which include: fear of hurting patients during examinations, anxiety about causing embarrassment and concern (and therefore avoidance) about discussing sensitive issues.

What do we know about palliative care patients' and carers' involvement with training of HPs?

As a result of the (National Institute of Clinical Excellence) NICE guidance on palliative and supportive care, there has been a concerted effort in the UK to increase communication skills training. It is likely that, in the future, all senior HPs in palliative care and oncology will be expected to gain an accredited qualification in communication skills.

It is hoped that patients will play an active role in this process; indeed, many strategic health planning groups and committees now have active involvement from an expert patient or user. The patients in this situation will usually have received some training themselves.

Formal assessment (for example in undergraduate and postgraduate examinations) of communication skills by simulated (actor) patients is now in widespread use in many countries including the UK. The use of actual 'patient-examiners' to assess communication skills of palliative care professionals is, however, still some way off. Although use of 'patient-examiners' might be a desirable aim, it may be difficult to achieve, because many patients may feel too ill and fatigued to participate in formal examinations. However, with the recent changes in medical and nursing training, it is likely that patients' feedback after consultations will form an increasingly important part of assessing the performance of palliative care professionals.

Hospice patients have not traditionally been involved in the teaching of basic examination and history-taking skills. However, a pilot study in a hospice in Leicester has suggested that this would be feasible, although there was concern from some of the nursing staff that very ill patients 'should not have their privacy invaded'. In addition to learning clinical skills, the students developed increased confidence in broaching sensitive issues: there was no evidence that the students were disadvantaged at the end of year assessments. Furthermore, 91% of the patients involved stated that they enjoyed teaching, and 95% were willing to repeat their involvement.[11]

There are anecdotal reports in the literature of individual students' experiences with meeting patients from hospices. In one such report a medical student met a woman of 84 with a chronic, incurable infection who was admitted to the hospice. He describes his discussions with her as 'one of the most powerful experiences I have had as a medical student.'

He learns about her hopes and expectations of recovery and further treatment options, and why she sometimes appears to contradict herself. On one occasion she states she has 'no reason to live' because she has no surviving family, while on another she has high hopes of a new treatment working for her. He concludes that this is because her condition fluctuates, and because she is a resilient person who 'endured two world wars and the Depression'. He also acknowledges the need, '... to relate better with patients with whom I have nothing in common', and that, 'I spent most of my time ... trying to persuade the patient to make what I believed to be the right choice. I now realise that the right choice is determined entirely by the patient.'[12]

This powerful lesson – the importance of treating every person as an individual – echoes the words of Dame Cicely Saunders, founder of the modern hospice movement: '... we are concerned both to relieve suffering and that our patients should maintain their own character and style to the end.'[13]

Internet-based learning

Web-based learning has a particular appeal in teaching communication skills for palliative care professionals, because patients' clinical conditions are often unstable: disease-related fatigue can have a huge impact on stamina, and therefore potential ability to teach or examine for long periods of time.

An excellent example of this method of teaching is demonstrated by the website known as 'The Database of Individual Patient Experiences' (Dipex).[14] This was co-founded by two doctors, one of whom had had personal experience of cancer.

There are taped audio and video recordings, with patients living with serious illnesses such as cancer. Users of the website can listen to, or watch clips of recordings, which are split into sub headings.

An interview with a woman with bowel cancer included 2 clips entitled '... information is important because it allows me to work with the medical team', and 'I was shocked when the consultant gave me bad news, and then said he had the wrong notes by mistake.'

Another woman with lymphoma and heart failure recorded an interview that included the following clips; '... the hospice is a happy, loving place where I've learned to write poetry', and 'acceptance is a great thing because it heals the mind.'

For each illness there are interviews with several people and, as a result, the reader can appreciate the broad range of reactions and coping mechanisms, which can occur when someone is diagnosed with a serious illness. Websites like this add to our teaching tools, particularly in the area of communication skills.

The 'goldfish bowl'

The 'goldfish bowl' is a teaching method, which has been developed principally to teach communication skills. The room is set up such that there is an inner circle of people including a facilitator, surrounded by a larger outer circle of people who are the 'observers'. People in the inner circle discuss the issues, while being listened to by the observers. The purpose of arranging the circles thus, is to provide a non-threatening atmosphere: the people in the inner circle have their backs to the outer. It has been used to teach undergraduates and postgraduates, but most often the 'teachers' in the inner circle are actors or fellow students who are role-playing.[15]

This teaching technique has been successfully adapted to teach final year medical students in a number of hospices in south-east England, since circa 2000. Each of the 4 hospices involved run 3–6 goldfish bowls per year, with 10–25 students attending each time. The success of these sessions is due largely to the teachers in the 'inner circle' who tend to be hospice day-care patients. The programme is reported by Edmonds and Burman.[16]

Patients attending day centre in the few weeks prior to each goldfish bowl are given an explanation of how the teaching is organised, and given the opportunity to get involved. During each session, the 'inner circle' consists of between 4 and 5 patients and a facilitator; the outer circle is the group of medical students – the 'observers'. The content of the goldfish bowl discussions are confidential and the students are asked to respect this.

The facilitator asks the patient group a series of open questions: individual patients respond if they feel comfortable to do so. Examples of questions include:

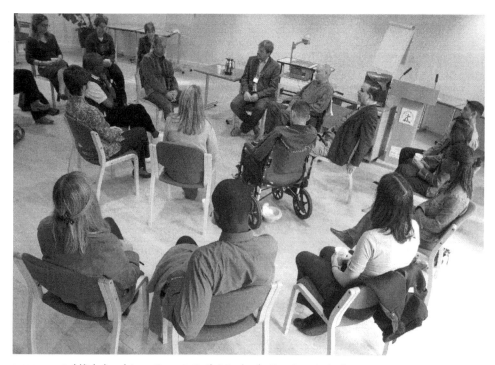

FIGURE 13 Goldfish bowl in action at St Christopher's Hospice, Sydenham.

▓ when someone first suggested you attended the hospice day centre what did you think?

▓ what do you get out of attending the day centre?

▓ what sort of therapies have you accessed since you have attended?

▓ can you tell us about your experiences as an in-patient either in the hospital or here in the hospice?

▓ can you tell us something about your experiences with doctors and nurses in the hospital or hospice?

Some key examples of useful insights from the patients about the experience of being diagnosed with a serious illness include:

▓ dispelling myths about hospices. 'Before I came to the day centre at the hospice I was terrified … I mean I'd always thought of hospices as somewhere you go and don't come out …' and 'I'd always thought hospices were just for people with cancer' (this from a patient with motor neurone disease)

▓ lessons learned from communication with health professionals. Some patients described positive experiences where news had been conveyed sensitively and, more importantly, tailored to them as an individual: 'I mean some people like it straight down the line don't they? … but I'm the sort of person that doesn't like to know everything at once'. Others described less helpful encounters: 'I mean he obviously hadn't bothered to read my notes before I went in …' and 'I don't feel I was properly warned about how awful chemotherapy was … if I'd known I might not have gone through with it'

▓ the atmosphere and range of therapies available in the day centre. Patients often described how they had surprised themselves and their carers by producing, for example, artwork and pieces of creative writing. Very often they had never undertaken such activities before. Others talked of the benefits of accessing complementary therapies and the beneficial effects on relaxation and pain. With regard to the atmosphere in the day centre, people talked about the feeling of solidarity amongst day centre attendees: 'You know there are other people in the same boat to talk to, but we don't just talk doom and gloom – it's a very happy place actually'. There is also a sense of learning from each other: 'We might all have cancer but we are all different and have all had different experiences of chemotherapy'

▓ the effects of illness on carers. 'My wife does everything for me … I come here partly to give her a break, and she's reassured that I'm being looked after on that day and she can relax and go out shopping'.

At the end of each session, patients are asked to give a 'take-home message' for the students, and the students then have the opportunity to direct questions to the patients, via the facilitator. Some examples of 'take-home messages' include:

▓ the importance of honesty and openness

▓ treating everyone as an individual

▓ taking time to understand how much information each patient would like.

Evaluation of the goldfish bowl by students

The sessions are usually evaluated highly by the students: in Edmonds and Burman's report, average scores from 23 hospice visits made by 242 students were between 5 and 5.6 (where the maximum score for each question was 6) for questions about clarity, relevance, information being pitched at the right level and overall usefulness.[16] These students were all undergraduates from a large medical school in South-East and Central London.

One of the participating hospices (Trinity Hospice), also uses the goldfish bowl to teach medical students on the graduate entry programme at St Georges's Hospital Medical School in South-West London: a total of 37 students provided feedback in June 2005.[17] The following themes emerged as learning points for the students:

* the importance of tailoring information to individual patient needs
* remembering that each patient is unique and individual
* need for honesty and openness
* importance of body language in communication
* where possible, give the patient the impression that you have all the time in the world
* impact of diagnosis and illness on whole family and carers
* the importance of dignity.

The students have experienced a variety of different teaching methods during their training, and were asked for specific feedback on this teaching method. Compared with other teaching methods, students rated the goldfish bowl very highly:

* it was the real thing – having worked so much with actors, I had to keep reminding myself these were real people
* I thought it would be intimidating, but that didn't seem to be a problem
* I was impressed that patients felt able to talk openly about personal issues.

Students were also asked to describe what they thought the potential benefits and difficulties this teaching method might raise for the patients. Benefits highlighted included:

* they are helping to shape the practice of future doctors
* participants seemed to enjoy the experience and appreciate being able to give something back
* therapeutic
* patients seemed comfortable and willing to share their experiences
* good to tell their story
* I hope they feel they have shaped our attitudes.

Potential difficulties raised included:

* may raise unresolved issues
* overall enjoyable, but it appeared to be quite difficult for them at times to talk about distressing experiences
* painful – but hopefully they will realise how much we learn from them
* frightening initially, but rewarding
* potentially daunting
* surprised how open they were able to be in this setting.

Evaluation of goldfish bowl by the patients (teachers)
The patients are debriefed by the facilitator after the students have left the room. It is important to get direct feedback from the patients on their experience of being teachers in the goldfish bowl.

A sample of 6 sessions involving a total of 34 patients was audio-taped at St Christopher's Hospice. The feedback from the patients was universally positive.[18] In fact, several patients were keen to repeat their participation and have done so very effectively. Although some patients show evidence of distress when discussing difficult experiences during the actual session, very few appear to experience this on an ongoing basis.

Feedback from carers has not been specifically requested, although the authors know of no instances of concern expressed by carers following the goldfish bowl teaching sessions.

Learning from carers

An example of carer involvement in teaching programmes in hospices is outlined by Wee and Hillier.[19] The particular strength of this programme, is that it provides an opportunity for interprofessional learning at the undergraduate stage: carers discuss particular aspects of the care provided to them, and the person they are caring for, with undergraduate students in medicine, nursing and allied health professions. In palliative care, team-working is vital, and this programme introduces this concept at an early stage of HPs' careers.

Future directions for patient and carer participation in palliative care teaching

In conclusion, patients and carers clearly have a significant role and huge potential to be involved in both the education and examination of health professionals. There is no doubt that palliative care can learn from the experiences of other specialties such as mental health. Our experience of the goldfish bowl teaching method has shown us that patients are often very willing to be involved, and the impact can be incredibly powerful for the students.

However, how can we maximise the opportunity for hospice patients to be involved in teaching medical students and other health professionals? Clearly, the nature of the palliative care population needs to be acknowledged, and the potential impact of fatigue and other symptoms taken into consideration. This is essential both in the planning, and delivery of education programmes. We must ensure that 'patient-teachers' give fully informed consent for their involvement at all times, and that they are well prepared and debriefed appropriately.

If palliative care patients are to be asked to participate more widely in HP training, we perhaps need to be more creative: internet-based learning, video and audio-taped recordings have been explored briefly in this chapter and such resources provide exciting ideas for potential future development. These methods would allow us to maximise the potential of teaching materials and at the same time limit the demand on patients.

Another potential way to reduce the burden on the patient population may be to increase the involvement of carers in a variety of education programmes, as they have extremely valuable contributions to share.

The concept of interprofessional learning at undergraduate level is still in the early stages of development, and the palliative care setting seems an ideal one to promote this; multiprofessional team working is an essential prerequisite for providing excellent care. It seems logical that team-working skills are developed as early as possible in all HPs' careers, and this is an area for potential development.

Whether a selected group of palliative care patients may be able to receive formal training to become 'expert patients', who can then act as examiners, and more formal teachers, has yet to be fully explored. Remuneration for patients who train to become teachers in palliative care may also become an important issue for the future.

The majority of teaching methods used in palliative care training have not been validated and this is another area for potential future development. The long-term efficacy of teaching communication skills remains unknown: it is likely that HPs will require continued and differing ways of attaining and demonstrating such skills as they progress through their career pathways.

On a final note, every encounter with a patient should provide an opportunity for learning, regardless of the seniority or specialty of the HP. It is only by truly listening to patients and regarding them as inspirational teachers that we can understand what is important to them and their carers. As Dame Cicely Saunders said:[20]

> Discussion of palliative treatments and competent symptom control can open up communication and bring support at a deep level … however, no report can take the place of an attentive listener and response to the questions an individual patient is asking at a particular time.

Jennifer Todd has been working as a part time consultant in palliative medicine at Trinity Hospice for 5 years having completed her specialist training on the South Thames Training Scheme. Her main areas of interest are teaching and training, professional development and ethics. She is currently involved in a wide range of teaching of healthcare professionals and finds the contribution of service users in education extremely valuable and powerful.

Emma Hall qualified in medicine from St George's Hospital in 1993. She trained in palliative medicine under the South Thames training scheme and commenced her first consultant post at St Christopher's Hospice, Sydenham in 2003. She has been involved in the training of medical students from the Guy's, King's and St Thomas's school of medicine since her appointment and is particularly interested in the expertise of service users as educators of future health professionals.

CHAPTER 13

The Tuesday group: a project in the art of dying

Sue Eckstein and Bobbie Farsides

Introduction

This chapter explores the reasons for, and process of, producing a play based on notes taken at a patient support group in an English hospice. The play realistically represents the conversations dying patients have with one another. The playwright and the academic who commissioned the piece worked together to produce a play which would reflect reality and inform those with a professional interest in care of the dying whilst at the same time making the experience of dying patients accessible to an audience untouched by the academic literature or practical experience.

The Tuesday group

Opening the box

Bobbie Farsides

On Saturday 22 February 2003, my friend and colleague Sue Eckstein and I spent a slightly surreal but wonderfully rewarding day in the company of a cast of professional actors. They had assembled to rehearse and perform a reading of *The Tuesday Group*, a play Sue had written at my request.

By the end of 2001, I was approaching the end of my time as director of a three-year project, funded by the European Commission, entitled 'European Palliative Care: ethics and communication'. The project had brought together a very experienced multidisciplinary team of palliative care professionals from Britain, Italy, Spain and the Netherlands, and our enquiries had ranged over a broad number of ethical issues relating to communication at the end of life. We had also embraced a broad range of methodologies, including systematic literature reviews, quantitative analysis of epidemiological data, qualitative analysis of focus group discussions, and more traditionally analytical/theoretical work on the underlying philosophical issues.

Our concerns had been various. We wanted to know how, if at all, communication practices across Europe were informed by a good understanding of the ethical issues around truth-telling and disclosure. We had looked at how differences in culture might explain and sometimes (though not always) justify radical differences in approach. And following on from this, we wanted to see if we could demonstrate any particular advantages attached to specific forms and manners of communication.

As the project drew to a close, we were painfully aware that one voice was missing from our enquiry, that of service users, which in this case meant terminally ill and dying patients. This was not a simple oversight on our part. We had considered various ways in which to pull in the patients' perspective, but some were beyond our resources and others had been rejected for ethical and/or methodological reasons. We were also aware of excellent work that we did not feel the need to replicate.[1,2,3] However, we could not accept that the project would be complete until we had given the users a voice in some way.

Quite early on in the project, Barbara Monroe, Chief Executive of St Christopher's Hospice in London and a project partner, had suggested that we look at a set of notes that the hospice had kept of meetings held within their day centre. The notes covered a period of ten years, and offered an account of discussions that took place within the context of the patient support group, facilitated by a hospice social worker. As such they gave a unique insight into the ways in which terminally ill patients communicated with one another when afforded a safe and structured environment in which to do so.

I remember spending two warm summer days immersed in the notes, taking in the personalities, the concerns and the patterns of interchange. I felt I got to know some people rather well as they attended the group over a period of time and contributed to discussions over a broad range of themes. Some people drove me mad, others I missed desperately when they 'disappeared', yet others remained mysterious and shadowy throughout. At the end of the process I knew that the notes held much that was valuable, but I also began to worry that it would be inappropriate to use them for the purpose I had in mind.

The initial intention had been to use the transcripts as the basis for a piece of substantive qualitative research, from which we would publish 'results'. We hoped to reveal and explore dominant themes and issues that arise when dying people talk to one another. Detailed discussions had taken place between myself and members of the hospice staff to decide the terms upon which such research could proceed. There was a significant amount of enthusiasm for the idea, with professionals involved in the group, past and present, seeing the value of revealing the data to a wider audience. However, on reflection there were a number of obstacles to this route:

- the notes were written by the social workers responsible for facilitating the groups and did not, as such, offer a verbatim account of the conversations held. Although the facilitators were experienced practitioners who understood the context within which they were operating and the clients with whom they were dealing, this would still be a problem when analysing the data. There were also differences in style and content reflecting which particular social worker had facilitated the group. This was interesting in and of itself, but probably told one more about the social workers than about the participants
- although participants' consent had been acquired, and this covered the use of the transcripts for teaching and/or research purposes, I did not feel that the nature of consent given permitted close analysis and verbatim quoting from the data. Because of a prior decision not to utilise any of the transcripts recorded within the preceding two years, retrospective consent could not be sought from participants. This concern fed in to a much larger current debate about the use of case study material in teaching and research, and it was felt that over-caution was preferable in this context[4]
- a primary and complex concern was in regard to confidentiality and anonymity. As healthcare professionals and/or researchers one could feel a duty of confidentiality

in a number of different ways:
- a duty of confidentiality owed to the dead
- a duty of confidentiality as owed to the living, which could include patients and/or families and significant others.

As mentioned above, living patients would effectively be protected by our decision not to include notes from groups held within the last two years. However, patients now deceased might still deserve to remain anonymous and their views confidential, particularly as what would be reported was a third-hand account of their views, which they would not be able to clarify or refute. Given the sensitive nature of the subjects discussed, there was also the worry of how belated recognition of what their loved ones were saying, thinking and experiencing might impact on their survivors. Families and friends might recognise themselves and/or their dead relations, despite attempts to secure anonymity; yet attempts to secure anonymity could potentially dilute the veracity of the data.

Hospice staff were particularly concerned about the effects of any research on existing group members and professionals, as well as on the future success of the group. I strongly endorsed and shared this concern. All the available evidence suggested the group discussions offered an effective and highly valued therapeutic benefit to participants, and nothing could be allowed to threaten this. We could not afford to put people off coming in future, nor did we want to negatively affect the experience of those currently attending.

Having acknowledged these issues, and having sought the advice of Local Research Ethics Committee chairs, I decided that analysis should not proceed. However, I was left feeling that it was unethical to return the transcripts to the box in which they had sat for the preceding years without attempting to give a public voice to the participants of the groups. I could not help feeling that what happened in these groups was a wonderful by-product of openness and honest communication. These people knew they were dying; doctors had told them so if they had not already worked it out for themselves. Now they were coming together to share time and conversation, and take from the group whatever they needed to make their experience more bearable. I wanted to offer this experience up for consideration, given what we had learnt about practices in other parts of Europe which were based on a belief that the truth (that someone was dying) was just too hard to bear, and no good would come of sharing it.

When thinking about how to get the voices heard, the research group was fortunate in three regards. First, at an early project meeting our Italian collaborators had made us aware of the work being done in their country to use the humanities to assist in discussing and theorising around death and dying. This development was echoed within the UK with a demonstrable development of the interface between the humanities, social science and medicine. My own institution, King's College London, had recently appointed the first Chair of Humanities in Medicine, and throughout 2002/3 was to be hosting a series of events on 'The Art of Dying'. To quote the brochure, this was 'a series of events in which scholars of the humanities, clinicians and social scientists investigate changing perspectives on what constitutes a good death across time and in a variety of cultures.'

Secondly, there had also been a significant development of what I had called in an earlier piece, *cancer narratives*.[5] These accounts made the ordinary extraordinary because of the way in which the authors chose to make their experience of disease public. Some writers already enjoyed high public profiles and then became celebrities because they were dying. Others were private individuals who, when faced with a life threatening disease or a terminal diagnosis, found the courage to share the experience with people they would never meet or know.[6,7,8,9,10,11,12,13] Whilst not wishing to underestimate the importance of these contributions, the St Christopher's notes represented something very different. They let us in to the private world of dying patients who were speaking to one another and not to an 'audience'.

Finally, St Christopher's Hospice was attempting to lead the way in terms of user involvement in the development of palliative care policy and provision of care. This was never going to be an easy task, but this project seemed to complement this broader aim. We hoped that we could bring the voices of former patients/service users into the debate and thereby add to the contributions made by those patients who were so generously contributing to the process of service evaluation and improvement.[14]

Perhaps our biggest piece of good fortune when looking for the way to give the patients a voice, was that we had amongst us a playwright willing to utilise the transcripts to create a piece of drama. What is more, she was willing to work within unusual constraints that meant her creative imagination could not be given full rein. The notes already laid out a drama of sorts, but the full nature of that particular drama could not, and would not, be revealed. Nor could we create new types of drama absent in the notes. What we needed to do was capture the essence, make the experience recognisable to those who were, or had been, a part of something similar, and open the experience up to those who may not even know such groups exist. We wanted to help the professionals caring for dying patients gain further insight, and we wanted to help to demystify the dying process and the dying patient for tomorrow's doctors and nurses. We wanted to produce a 'true' but fictional account, something real which appropriately reflected what we had found in the box of notes.

It was therefore decided to use the transcripts to inform, inspire and shape a piece of dramatic writing – a decision we felt happy with in the light of the concerns expressed above.[15,16,17,18,19,20] At first we saw this play being used in the hospice and in the classroom, but as I revealed at the beginning of this piece, it very soon found a more public stage.

Opening the curtains

Sue Eckstein

What is particularly missing from stories, films and plays about death is the experience of hearing ordinary people who are dying talking to each other. It was only when I accepted this commission that I began to understand why this could be!

My brief was very specific: I had to use the reports as a primary source of information and turn them into a work of fiction. The play had to accurately reflect the content of the reports and the environment in which the meetings took place. It also had to be of interest to a wide and general audience as well as medical students and palliative care professionals.

I kept a diary while I wrote the play. The early entries reflect the complexity of the task, my initial reservations and my growing excitement.

5 October 2001

Bobbie kneels on the carpet; piles of paper in folders surround her. These are the transcripts of a series of meetings of groups of people who are dying. There is something almost unbearable in the knowledge that all the people who made up these groups are now dead. I wonder aloud how we could use their experience so that their voices can have a wider resonance, without exploiting them or trespassing on their privacy. Bobbie thinks it can be done. Knowing that confidentiality is one thing that Bobbie is very clear about, and committed to, makes me feel that it might be possible. We agree that she will anonymise the transcripts further before I read them myself. So far, I don't have any firm ideas of what I will do with the information. I like the idea of a mixture of dialogue and interior monologue and I like the idea of it not being immediately clear what the group is meeting for.

15 October 2001
I have read through most of the transcripts very fast, reading to get a feel for the kinds of things that were said rather than to build up a detailed picture of how each group functioned. I am struck by the fact that I have never read anything like this – that we so rarely hear the words of the terminally ill except on death beds in novels and what a valuable resource it is. I am struck too by the amount of crying that goes on in the groups – how to dramatise that and make it bearable to listen to?

9 November 2001
On Thursday, Bobbie and I visited St Christopher's Hospice and had a meeting with Barbara Monroe and the Director of Social Work, Isobel Bremner. It was agreed that the resource we had should be treasured and not wasted. We talked a lot about confidentiality. I made it very clear that I would be inventing characters to voice the main themes and that no one would be identifiable. It seems significant that I am not using transcripts of what people said but of a social worker's impressions of what was said and what happened. We spent some time in the day centre. There was something extraordinarily moving about being in the actual room where all those meetings had taken place. In the corridor we passed a little boy, chattering happily, being led by the hand by a member of staff. I didn't know anything about him, why he was there or who he was visiting, but I felt a lump in my throat. Bobbie noticed the effect the child had on me, and said later that she was not sure whether to share her suspicion that he had been working on a memory box for his mother or father. I keep seeing the image of this little boy. I wonder why I should be so moved by it. Maybe it is because it is quite easy to detach from what goes on in hospitals where there is the intention, or at least the hope, that patients will get better and leave. It is hard to detach from a hospice. At any time in the future, that little boy could be my own son or daughter.

After the visit to the hospice, I re-read the reports and, in no particular order, noted down all the key issues. These included: groups and group dynamics, the reactions of others, anger/irritation, men and women's differences, marriage, children, physical symptoms/illness, life choices/changes, religion/faith, death and general chat/gossip.

I decided that I would need eight group members, each of whom would have their own distinct personalities and life stories, and who would allow all these issues to be raised. The characters needed to reflect both the demography of the area in which the hospice was situated and the typical make-up of hospice discussion groups as suggested by the transcripts and corroborated by Barbara Monroe.

The catchment area of St Christopher's has a well-established black community, so I created George, seventy-three, a Jamaican who came over to Britain on the SS *Windrush* in 1948 and has lived here ever since, and Josie who is thirty-four and of West African origin. She is bringing up her seven-year-old daughter alone.

I wanted to show that many people living with terminal illness have a dual role – that of patient *and* carer, so I created Margaret. She is in her late seventies and has been a housewife and mother all her life. She is married to Jack who is also ill with cancer. She has decided not burden her husband with the knowledge of her cancer.

Then I wanted two women in their forties who would be typical of the sorts of people who might be attracted to a group of this kind: Mary is a paediatric nurse who lives with her husband and fifteen-year-old son. Rachel has three young children and a husband who is a documentary producer. She is an illustrator and writer of children's books.

In contrast to Mary and Rachel, I needed a character who would be profoundly uncomfortable in a discussion group such as this one: Catherine, sixty, is single and has no children. She is a retired teacher who has no close family or friends to support her.

For many people, terminal illness is just one of the many difficult and painful things going on in their lives: sixty-six year old Vi had been a school cook before stopping work to look after her husband who had Alzheimer's and who has recently died. Her very difficult daughter and four grandchildren under eight have moved into her one bedroom flat. One of her other children was killed in a motorcycle accident when he was eighteen.

And then there is Dan who is in his early twenties. He is a film and music enthusiast who lives at home with his parents and his pet fire belly toad and rat.

Having created my characters, I did a second re-ordering of the material, allocating phrases or themes to individuals. This allocation turned out to be quite fluid, as the characters developed their own distinct personalities. I produced a plan of the five weeks and worked out who would be present in which group and roughly what they would talk about. This, too, turned into a fluid exercise. Dan was due to appear in only one group but seemed keen to come in for a second week. I intended that Catherine should say very little throughout the play but gradually she got drawn into the action and found her voice. Rachel, on the surface the most articulate member of the group, turned out to be the quickest to make false assumptions about people. I had always planned for Mary to find the father she had never known, but had never planned for the sudden death of Margaret's grandson. I had always understood the relationship between Rachel and her children but had never planned that Josie's daughter should have been adopted.

Writing a play to a very tight brief such as this one is an unusual task, and not without its difficulties. Throughout the process there was considerable tension between the need to make the play reflect the workings and preoccupations of the groups at the hospice and the need to make it work as a piece of dramatic art that could stand up on its own. For example, although we knew from the transcripts there would rarely be young people in the groups, I decided that for dramatic purposes, my group would include two characters under thirty-five. This was the first of the decisions I had to make about the conflict between accuracy and dramatic effect. It was felt that this was an acceptable decision and one which would not compromise the veracity of the piece.

There were other instances, however, where it would have been both unethical and unreasonable to deviate from the 'reality' of the transcripts for dramatic effect. Conflict – such as that between individual group members, or (better still) the convenor and the group members, or violent outbursts and chair-throwing – may have made for exciting drama but did not reflect the reality of the groups which was of tolerance, growing compatibility, and support. So when a literary manager of a London theatre commented on an early version of the play that 'Laura [the social worker and group convenor] remains responsible, reliable and receptive and so is less interesting and complex as a dramatic character than I think she might be (no discernible tension is generated by her relationship to and difference from the group)', I did not feel that it would be right to make the changes that were suggested.

I proposed at the outset that I would discuss the first draft of each of the five episodes with Bobbie Farsides, whose comments and suggestions I then incorporated in the second draft of each episode. The first draft of the complete play was shown to Barbara Monroe and Isobel Bremner. I received some very helpful feedback from them, particularly on how Laura, the social worker, might manage the group and relate to the other characters. For example, I needed their experience to know under what circumstances Laura would leave the room with a distraught group member, how far she would direct the members' conversations and whether, for example, she would allow individuals to flout rules if it meant they would remain in the group.

Quite by chance, one of my characters turned out to have an uncanny resemblance to a group member who had recently died. This was not something that either Bobbie or I could have been aware of without input from hospice staff. I was able to change various aspects of my character's life so that there would be no danger that relatives would be offended or upset.

When I started to give the characters voices, I thought it would be necessary to know what cancer or other illness they were suffering from and what the physical symptoms would be. I spent several evenings on the Cancer Bacup website before realising that I did not need to have this information to bring the characters alive. I was, however, careful to ensure that the few medical facts I did use were correct. For example, I asked a pharmacist friend what colour the capsule of a particular dose of morphine would be.

The reports of group meetings referred to periods of silence and to participants sometimes choosing to say very little. I had to find a way of portraying silence and the places to which people go when they distance themselves from the proceedings. I used interior monologues to allow characters to 'leave the group'.These monologues also allowed the characters a life outside the confines of the room.

CATHERINE:	I think I'll stick with aromatherapy.
MARGARET:	I've heard that's very nice. But imagine what Jack would think if I came home smelling of roses and lavender and …
	(Voices fade. Conversations continue in the background.)
	(A clifftop. Sound of wind and gulls.)
VI: *(Voice over)*	And round our caravan there'd be flowerbeds marked out with white-painted pebbles. And we'd grow those old-fashioned roses. And between them, Eddie would plant lavender and violets and forget-me-nots and we'd watch the bees and butterflies and Eddie would squeeze my hand and say 'forget-me-not, Violet, forget-me-not.' And at night we'd lie with our arms around each other and when the wind died down and the sea calmed we'd listen to the sound of each other's hearts beating.
	(Vi's voice fades.)
	(Back to Day Centre where the conversation has been continuing.)
MARGARET:	Oh no. I'm far too old for cosmetic surgery. The face-lift would outlive the face by a long way. And Jack gets confused enough as it is without me suddenly coming home looking like Marlene Dietrich.
CATHERINE:	No. Aromatherapy. They do it in here, you know.
MARGARET:	I don't know about all this alternative medicine. It's never been properly tested – not like the drugs you're given by the doctor.

CATHERINE: Well, if all it does is make me feel a bit better for a couple of hours, that's more than I can say for most of the chemicals they pump into me. I can really recommend black pepper aromatherapy for constipation. It's changed my life.

GEORGE: I'd try anything short of getting Dynorod out. And I've even considered that once or twice I can tell you!

I originally thought of using poetry as another device to represent silence in the group, with Catherine 'disappearing' into memories of poems sparked by a single thought or word. I found that the poems in her head added another dimension – almost another character – to the play. I intentionally did not use the more recognisable 'death poems' by poets such as Sylvia Plath and Emily Dickinson. I wanted the audience to listen to the words rather than be distracted by remembering where they had last read or heard the poems, so I used less well-known but very powerful poems by writers such as Anne Sexton, Stevie Smith, Jon Silkin and Denise Levertov, and extracts by Virginia Woolf – not from Mrs Dalloway or A Room of One's Own, but from one of her essays 'On Being Ill' from *The Crowded Dance of Modern Life.*

> We do not know our own souls, let alone the souls of others. Human beings do not go hand in hand the whole stretch of the way. There is a virgin forest in each; a snowfield where even the print of birds' feet is unknown. Here we go alone, and like it better so. Always to have sympathy, always to be accompanied, always to be understood would be intolerable.

When reading the reports, and sorting out themes, I was surprised at how little the really big issues, such as death and disease, dominated the conversations and how important everyday concerns and 'trivia' were. This 'trivia' had to be given the same importance as the other, more immediately weighty, topics. Participants in the groups were not shut off from the world – they frequently commented on national and international events, so it was important that, in the play, current affairs were reflected in signs and signifiers. For instance, characters talk about the Harry Potter phenomenon, bargains at well-known department stores, the increasing use of cosmetic surgery by celebrities.

I was also surprised, when I finished writing the play, at how much humour there was in it, and how the mood could swing from joy to sadness and back again very quickly. Listening to the recording of the performance of the play, the audience's laughter, triggered by the immaculate comic timing of the actors, infiltrates almost every scene:

CATHERINE: Why do we do it – all this quiet, polite suffering? There's something to be said for brain tumour disinhibition, you know. Apparently, when I was an in-patient last year, I said to one of the nurses: 'I don't know how you can live with yourself with an arse like that.'
               (*Laughter – George coughs.*)

MARGARET: Ooh, you didn't!

CATHERINE: I taught English at the girls' grammar school for nearly forty years. And, you know, so much of what has been written – so much of the really beautiful poetry and prose – has been written by people suffering out loud.

VI: 'The Daffodils'. Now that's what I call really beautiful and there's no suffering in it anywhere as far as I can remember.

'I wandered lonely as a cloud that floats on high o'er vale and hill—'
I'm sure I used to know more of it than that. Must be these drugs.

MARGARET: There's lots of beautiful poetry without suffering in it. What about Patience Strong?

CATHERINE: Patience Strong?!

GEORGE: Careful now, Catherine my darling. We don't want you choking too. Poor Laura's looking nervous enough with me in the room.

CATHERINE: 'Elegy for a still-born child', by Seamus Heaney. There's beauty in that suffering.

> 'On lonely journeys I think of it all,
> Birth of death, exhumation for burial,
> A wreath of small clothes, a memorial pram,
> And parents reaching for a phantom limb.'

(Silence. Someone sniffs.)

RACHEL: That must be the worst thing, I think. Losing a child.

(Laura passes Vi a tissue.)

LAURA: Here, Vi.

(Vi wipes her eyes and blows her nose. Silence.)

RACHEL: At least the group feels safe. I can just be who I am. And I don't have to try to make things feel better for anyone. *(Pause)* You know, Mike can only go to sleep if he's asked me if I'm still fighting and I've said yes. And then he goes to sleep and I lie there thinking about what'll happen when I get too sick to look after the children.

CATHERINE: My sister doesn't believe you can't beat a brain tumour. And whatever I've got, she's sure to have had something worse and made a full recovery. If I tell her that her bronchitis isn't in quite the same league, she goes into a frightful sulk and her visits become even rarer. No great loss, really. It's been a long time since I came anywhere near the salukis in her affections.

GEORGE: Now am I being stupid, Catherine, or are you saying your sister's got a thing for Japanese engineering?

CATHERINE: *(Laughs)* Salukis. They're pedigree dogs. Sort of hairy greyhounds with attitude. Goodness! That's the first time I've laughed in months. I've been feeling so terribly depressed.

RACHEL: 'Noble deeds and hot baths are the best cures for depression.' Dodie Smith, I think.

GEORGE: When I couldn't get into my bath any more, the lovely OT put in a hoist but the district nurse was used to a different make and couldn't work out how to use it.

LAURA: She should have got back to the OT.

GEORGE: Well, we'd just sit and have a nice cup of tea together instead.

VI: Sounds like heaven to me.

Although at the outset of the project we had had no plans for the play to be performed, King's College's Art of Dying symposium provided the perfect opportunity to showcase *The Tuesday Group*. With tremendous support from St Christopher's Hospice, a professional director was taken on and the play was cast. We were privileged to have a cast of well-known and hugely talented actors – Gina McKee, Phyllida Law, Sarah Collier, Will

Godfrey, Candida Gubbins, Stefan Kalipha, Jacqueline Kington, Amanda Mealing and Jean Trend.

It was really heartening to receive positive feedback about the play from the actors when they arrived for the rehearsal. This was the first confirmation we had had that the play could genuinely appeal to those with no professional interest in the subject matter. We were both moved and gratified that one of the actors, who was herself undergoing chemotherapy for recently diagnosed breast cancer, felt that so much of the script echoed her thoughts and feelings.

The cast's enthusiasm was echoed by an audience of over 300 people. Even now, over three years later, we are still receiving requests for copies of the script and permission to use the play both within a hospice setting and in a wider context.

Whatever happens to *The Tuesday Group* next, I feel proud and privileged to have been involved in this unique and very special project.

Acknowledgments

We would like to thank the European Commission for funding the project; Barbara Monroe and the staff of St Christopher's Hospice, Sydenham for giving us this opportunity; and the participants, past and present of the St Christopher's Patient Support Group.

This work was funded by the European Commission Grant BMH4-CT98–3881 *European Palliative Care: Ethics and Communication.*

Sue Eckstein studied drama at Walnut Hill School of Performing Arts, Massachusetts, USA on an English-Speaking Union Scholarship before going on to study English Literature at Durham University. She then taught in Sri Lanka where she was given a work permit on condition that she wrote a traditional pantomime for the school at which she taught. Three pantomimes later, she returned to the UK where she joined Voluntary Service Overseas (VSO) and worked as a programme manager in Bhutan and The Gambia, and devised, set up and managed VSO's Overseas Training Programme. In 1999, she joined the Centre of Medical Law and Ethics, King's College London where she is currently Director of Programme Development, specialising in ethical issues in medical research.

Now living in Brighton, Sue co-wrote and produced the *Mrs Hoover Show* which was performed at the Komedia Theatre, and studied creative writing at Sussex University. She was awarded a post-graduate diploma in dramatic writing and an MA in Creative Writing, The Arts and Education. Her play, *Kaffir Lilies*, was broadcast on BBC Radio 4 in July 2006.

Bobbie Farsides has been teaching and researching in the field of bioethics for almost twenty years. She has a long-standing interest in the ethical issues relating to death and dying and whilst at Keele University set up the first specialist MA in the Ethics of Cancer and Palliative Care in conjunction with Marie Curie Cancer Care. When she moved to

King's Collge London she forged strong links with both the Department of Palliative Care and Policy at Guy's, King's and St Thomas's Medical School and St Christopher's Hospice, Sydenham. These collaborations led to a European Commission funded project looking at Ethics and Communication in European Palliative Care, which in turn led to the writing of *The Tuesday Group* play. Bobbie served as a Specialist Advisor to the House of Lords Select Committee on the Assisted Dying and Terminal Illness Bill and has recently been involved with the redrafting of the BMA's guidance on Withholding and Withdrawing Medical Treatment.

In July 2006 she moved to a new post at the Brighton and Sussex Medical School where she holds the Foundation Chair in Clinical and Biomedical Ethics. With her colleague and friend Sue Eckstein she co-edits the journal *Clinical Ethics*. Since starting her new job she has begun working closely with palliative care teams in the Sussex area, and is engaged in a project to involve the people of Brighton and Hove in more active discussions about living with the reality of dying.

CHAPTER 14

Voicing change: online not in line

Lucinda Jarrett

Introduction

In the year when MySpace helped to revolutionise the music industry and when Wikipedia, the free encyclopedia that anyone can edit, became more frequently used than Encyclopedia Britannica online, it would be foolish not to credit digital technology with transforming the way in which users get involved in production.

The chapters in this book show clearly that enabling individuals to find their creative voice gives them the confidence to get more involved in the delivery of care. In the second part of the book we have seen how support is critical in bringing groups together to build a collective voice that might deliver change. We have seen how the benefits of user involvement in arts practices are multiple both for individuals and groups: participants and carers may benefit from increased self-esteem, increased confidence and increased mental health. Carers may gain practical benefits, by learning new skills and gaining employment opportunities, for example.

Finding your voice can be an end in itself. However, in reality, most people seek user involvement because they believe some useful change will transpire. We have seen how support groups can nurture a collective voice without the idea of group action and political change being part of the agenda. Nor should they be. In the last sector of the book we have seen how services may benefit from better communication between users and staff – improvement on access to services and ward environments, for instance. The delivery of change in practice is not yet evidenced through widespread use of user involvement.

In this chapter I look at the potential of digital technology to be part of the strategy for the delivery of change in the future.

Website technology

The profile of MySpace.com rocketed overnight in July 2005 when News Corp paid £332.85m for parent company Intermix Media. At the time the move provoked derision because the company had no fixed assets it could sell. A year and several copycat deals later, it looks like a bargain. The Arctic Monkeys launched their single through MySpace.com, Lily Allen's album rocketed to Number 1 in the charts when it was launched on MySpace and digital downloads spearheaded the revolution in pop music sales.

The significance of this phenomenon is that all the content on both Wikipedia and MySpace is generated by users and it is uncensored. The founder of MySpace believes that the answer in driving access to new technology for the next generation lies not in webfilters, firewalls or censorship but in education. He has a point. We do not expect drivers to keep out of residential areas, but we do expect them to drive at 30mph and children to learn road safety and to use pedestrian crossings. With education, a user–led site can be encouraged to traffic useful information and encourage social networking between support groups locally and nationally.

MySpace has been criticised for poor webdesign, but actually it is this lack of production aesthetic that makes it approachable, easy to use and adaptable to individual taste. In June 2006 MySpace had 54 million unique users in the US. It has spearheaded new social networking sites, like Bebo, for school children and Facebook for university students and many more copycat sites, like Friendster and Tripod.

Can we use and adapt these for healthcare institutions and health providers? Most online social networking sites or user generated sites primarily provide information. When this content is made and uploaded by users, there is little one can do to guarantee accuracy, yet the healthcare community regard accuracy as essential. When people who are frail and vulnerable seek information and advice from the internet we assume there is a clear need for this to be definitive and accurate. Maybe we should challenge this assumption and recognise that there is a greater need for patients to participate in providing information to each other and to participate in sharing the progress of access to information.

Wikipedia is a good example. James Walley, its founder, has said that the content on the site should not be relied on for academic purposes but used for general reference. He suggests that Wikipedia should be seen as a 'work in progress'. I like this idea – a work that is constantly revisited, revised and updated and never be consulted as an absolute authority. With a team of 13 000 volunteers – that's you and me – editing 2.5billion pages, he says that the online encyclopaedia should be used for 'good solid background information'.

He refused to apologise to students who wrote to him complaining about F Grades for essays or class projects that cite Wikipedia as a source. 'For God's sake, you're at college, don't cite the encyclopaedia. If you are reading history at university, you should not be using a site with content generated by volunteers as a source, you should be reading history books,' he said at a conference at the University of Pennsylvania entitled 'The Hyperlinked Society' in June 2006.

Website innovation within healthcare

There are websites that have been set up to provide information for people living with cancer, www.promotingexcellence.org, www.dying.about.com for instance, but there are very few with user generated content for users. The website www.dipex.org provides medical narratives of illness and it is a fantastic and invaluable reference for doctors and/or patients. The site is a unique resource and one that will be extended to include 100 important diseases, as well as health related matters such as pregnancy screening, immunisation, children of parents with cancer and chronic illness, amongst others. The Dipex site is primarily a teaching resource aimed at health professionals designed to be reproduced and republished for distribution to GP surgeries, out-patient clinics, support groups, public libraries etc. The site also provides reliable information about illnesses and health issues like, What is Cancer? or What is the treatment for…? and there are answers to frequently asked questions and discussion of themes that have been raised during the interviews.

However, Dipex is not a reference source that can be constantly added and changed. It is therefore a site that is useful for hospice users to access but it offers only limited participation through some forums and the possibility that your narrative might be chosen to be published. It is driven by narratives recorded by researchers from hospice users but it does not directly invite user involvement. It is controlled by the researchers conducting the interview. Yet the strength of the digital revolution is in its ability to give control of the information and the means of production to the user and, in my view, this is the challenge for the hospice movement – to find ways of safely handing over control to the information provider of the information server or the website.

This is a shift from websites that are passive – like shop windows – to the Web 2 dynamic site that prompts and is dependent upon interaction from those using the site. The heart to this approach lies in seeing online information as a conversation. Message boards and online forums are highly useful for people who are often alone with their illness and not always able to confide or trust their worries to their families. An online conversation acts as a sounding board, a place where your worries can be aired and heard. This will never replace the GP or the doctor but it will often give people the confidence to express their fears to the doctor. Support groups provide a physical place where these worries and fears can be aired, but not all people living with illness can access a support group and online support could be significant for these communities.

Ten or fifteen years ago an online support network with user-generated and uploaded content would have been impossible. The technology was not there, nor was there the confidence in an open and uncensored exchange of information. Today, it is not only the technology revolution that is changing all this, but also the revolution in healthcare. HIV and AIDS transformed the way in which doctors and patients held and shared information. No one understood the illness and for the first time medical professionals found themselves facing patients who knew more about their illness and its treatment than they did. I worked with one young man who had nursed several friends as they died and saw the shattering of their hopes and lives when AZT failed them. He witnessed the introduction of combination therapies and waited two years until he felt confident about the science before going to his doctor and telling him exactly which medications he was prepared to take and why. He often found himself better informed than the doctors who were treating him and always made sure he had the most updated information available on all medication. With the help of the internet the patient's trust in the absolute authority of the medical professional was shaken by the onset of AIDS and this paradigm shift has helped drive the change towards greater user involvement in the delivery of holistic care.

The media revolution

The digital revolution has paralleled the healthcare revolution and influenced an agenda for greater patient access to the technologies of media production and increased participation from the service user.

The filmmaking industry has been transformed by digital technology. For a start, the actual medium of film now barely plays a part, with the transition to digital tape and, latterly, solid state storage, now virtually complete. When I first worked in television in 1992, a film crew consisted of a director, a director's assistant, a cameraman, a cameraman's assistant, a sound recordist and a production team that included researchers, associate producers, an executive producer, and a director. Then there was post-production – weeks of expensive editing with an editor and a cutting room. The editor had his assistant, whose main job it was to supervise the mechanical numbering and classification of every last frame of celluloid, thereby assisting the manual editing process led by the editor. Then came the prints, and the grading, and the dub, and another print, and so on – a large scale and quite cumbersome division of labour that cost a lot of money and put filmmaking beyond the reach of all but the serious hobbyists with their Super 8 cameras and attic spaces. This situation has now changed completely, not only transforming the way television programmes and movies are made but putting movie making of a quality undreamt of even ten years ago within reach of everyone. Today, it's not an exaggeration to say that I can fit all the equipment required to make a programme of broadcast quality – video camera, microphone, laptop – into a stoutish shoulder bag. And the crew? That's just me. And the editor? Me again. The production team? What team!

The digital revolution reaches yet further. DVD authoring means that films can be mastered and duplicated from a laptop. Distribution can be managed through the internet. Even promotion is cheaper and easier to target. The feature film *The Blair Witch Project* was promoted through the internet and built an online fan base before it ever reached the screens.

These are huge developments. One, or at most two person crews, miniscule production costs, lightness and accessibility of equipment, immediacy and spontaneity, mean that filmmaking can be used more widely within palliative care and healthcare service delivery to enable service users to control the representation of their voice and its distribution.

The digital revolution within palliative care

Palliative care has not ignored the digital revolution. Many day centres now have computers and broadband access. At Rosetta Life we have made inroads into working with digital technology but are still some way off from realising its full potential.

In 1996 Rosetta Life began working in hospices, enabling those facing death to take control of the way in which they were represented by giving them the means to tell stories that had shaped their life experiences. The digital revolution was beginning to gain momentum. Digital cameras were affordable and simple non-linear editing software on computers enabled people to transcend the limitations of home movies.

The expansion of new media potential and the growth of patient involvement in healthcare and the new media revolution is exemplified by the story of two patients who worked with us in the early days of Rosetta Life. Garry Wall and David Graham both attended St John's Hospice in north west London and were working with us to gain skills in filmmaking. In 1998, using our cameras, computers, and know how they made a documentary entitled, *To a Future with Love* … the aim of which was to influence sexual health practice by reminding a younger gay generation who were becoming increasingly casual about sexual protection about the continuing dangers of HIV/AIDS. This new generation were not adult when the AIDS nightmare began and were convinced that the availability of combination therapy meant that HIV infection was no longer life-threatening. They filmed at three festivals and screened their movie widely within the gay community.

In 2001 Rosetta Life set up digital arts centres and broadband connections at ten hospices in England. The aim was to enable hospice users to find creative expression 'for what mattered' in the digital art form of their choice. The artwork belonged to the user, who was offered the basic skills by trained digital artists to make something of their life stories. Over the past five years we have seen many hospice users thrive in this approach to digital creativity. The process has had a profound effect on of the way that they are remembered, the way that they communicate to healthcare providers, the way in which they work with and engage with their immediate communities. Digital creativity enables the life threatened to regain some control over their lives, to be proud once again, to find meaning. Some of the stories of this process are told in this book.

At hospices where Rosetta Life artists work, artists train volunteers who are interested in new media work to deliver this support.

One of the key challenges of digital creativity is how far to open the doors to a wider online community. Closed communities are by definition limited but also safe. At Rosetta Life we are exploring ways of widening our community safely, through partnerships with the MS Society, the MND Associations and the Stroke Association. While anyone can visit our website, we have not yet created an interactive online community that is nationally accessible. Like all organisations seeking to develop appropriate models of new technology for healthcare we are constantly looking at what has already been developed elsewhere.

e-government: the future within palliative care

e-government is a model worth looking at. The digital revolution has been embraced by the government which has responded to the new media revolution with open government: meetings and minutes of local council meetings available online. Webcasts of strategy meetings and council meetings that used to be closed are now open to all who have access to downloading video. e-government has not only opened access to information but also made real differences to the housebound and the disabled who can vote and participate in local, regional and national politics from their laptops. This offers an interesting model for innovation within palliative care.

In response non-governmental organisations and lobbying groups have also found that new media forms such as email, blogs and texting have made it increasingly easier to disseminate information through the internet and has revolutionised the way in which lobbyists can campaign for policy change. We receive emails inviting us to sign our names to political campaigns that cover countless political issues from international questions, to climate change, developing world debt reduction and stop-the-war coalition, and local planning and neighbourhood issues. These campaigns make it easy for people to participate in political debate and make effective campaigning much inexpensive. Email lists can quickly gather thousands of names where before volunteers would have had to gather them laboriously on the doorstep.

This combination of popular access and governmental initiatives to increase access should have an impact on healthcare. A European parliament initiative demonstrates the potential impact of user participation in social care. In 2005 the Council of Europe published a paper entitled 'The role of new information technology as regards user involvement in Social Services'. Written by Francisco Gonzalez from University of Seville, the paper recommended that all public departments and agencies promote legal and political bases for the development of 'e-governance' in order to open up social services to user participation. The paper found that the opening up of social services was a key commitment of the Council of Europe, but that information and communications technology (ICT) could not be a genuine option without the support of local authorities and leadership from within communities. Without this support ICT would just be another form of social exclusion. The paper concluded:

> In order to develop participation by social service users in information, advice, consultation and co-operation activities, the parties directly involved must therefore agree on and accept in advance: the meaning of e-participation as empowerment [but] ... this will only work if we address the barriers that hospice users face with technology as well as the potential.

The same dilemma faces healthcare providers. People who are elderly and who have no continuous access to ICT cannot use the internet for access to information/webcasts/online social networking unless the means to teach ICT and provide assistance with installation of broadband and computer technology are made available.

The computer may remain a barrier for many but there is a drive to address this by using the more accessible medium of television for internet access. A simple attachment fitted to the back of the television can enable hospice users to use their remote controls to access the internet, send email, access online e-learning modules and download video and music from the internet. This may help the more frail overcome the physical barriers of access.

The future and its challenges – a personal perspective

It is easy to idealise the potential of new technology. 'It is great when it works' is the downfall of many new online initiatives. When the equipment does not work it is frustrating and people quickly become disheartened and disengaged. Webcasts may seem to offer an ideal opportunity to provide widespread access to events for people who are housebound enabling them to communicate with many people, but in reality people still prefer the telly to a computer. Internet communciation is still unpredictable and unreliable.

We ran a webcast from Trinity Hospice on World Hospice Day 2006. The concert had widespread publicity because Billy Bragg was releasing 'We Laughed', the song he had written with hospice user Maxine Edgington, in the UK charts. Sky TV broadcast a live interview with Billy and Maxine and BBC TV news interviewed another hospice user on the day of the concert. However, only 400 people logged onto the webcast despite the publicity while an audience of ten million watched the song performed live on BBC TV on New Year's Eve.

Moreover, the internet is still disturbingly slow and can substantially distort voice and image. A voice may travel from London via Hong Kong and Melbourne to reach Ipswich if that way is easiest for the information to flow and this creates surprising and unexpected delays. Many people use the free internet telephone system Skype for conversations but in practice when we used it to connect children from a South African hospice to the concert we held on World Hospice Day the distortion was so upsetting that Billy Bragg joked about the dawn of broadcasting and the first crackly days of television. While it is exciting to work with the pioneers of new technology and to engage those facing death with the potential of the new, we must be wary of disappointing.

I have set up web cam links between people in hospices and friends on the other side of the world that have been successful and remarkable, but I have also set up webcasts that have failed because the people got the time wrong or were late getting to an internet café because they couldn't park. We resorted to mobile phones to call them and felt foolish sitting in front of blank computer screens when the phones were so much more efficient. In fact, telephones do offer efficient interactivity and phone technologies are much underused. In rural Suffolk, where it is sometimes hard for people to reach the hospice for group support, a carers' group meeting takes place through telephone conferencing. Mobile phones can make group support a reality in rural areas.

At the Highland Hospice in Inverness, the medical staff are pioneering the use of PDA and mobile phones to enable hospice service users from outlying areas to become more involved and more connected with the delivery of their care. The medical team are developing a model for palliative care that was piloted in a study for chemotherapy patients by Stirling University. It enables patients to respond to questions via mobile phones that enable the monitoring of symptoms. If, for example, a person's temperature rises by a certain amount then patients are referred to online self-help. If the temperature rise becomes dangerous then the phone response goes direct to a medical professional who will contact the patient immediately. This use of technology is particularly appropriate for rural areas where it is both costly and difficult for patients to attend doctor's appointments. By enabling patients to monitor their own symptoms doctors can ensure immediate response and help patients to gain control over their delivery of care.

The mobile phone model could be adapted to enable social networking and creative projects to take place remotely and online. Last year we set up an online songmaking project, www.thesongrooms.org that provides children using paediatric palliative care from ten children's hospices across the world to write their own songs and share them. In Zimbabwe broadband connections are few and unpredictable so the children are using mobile phones as modems to upload recorded sound from their phones directly to the server. They can also upload text messages to vote for their most popular song and pictures and photos of their environment and their music workshops.

There is a real potential to combine online access to information with user generated creative content to create a social networking and information site for the palliative care community that will create a collective voice for service users in order to deliver practical change.

In the next ten years the most significant development in new technology will be 'web 3'/semantic technologies. Technologies that tell you what you need instead of you needing to request information. Based on information you input technologies will predict what you need and where to get it. It is currently particularly targeted at social networking: it will know who you want to meet and where they are. The implications are that websites will tell you what you need before you are aware of it yourself. If this kind of development becomes part of the mobile phone initiative being introduced at Highland Hospice, the mobile phone will send you the information you need and tell you where your nearest consultant is before you request it and could also send you information about available district nurses and other patients who might share collectively assimilated knowledge. In the context of the songmaking site for paediatric palliative care, a phone could send you information about where children are and when they want to make contact with you, prompting children who are often dispirited to communicate and connect and build friendships online.

The realisation of these ideas requires courage and strong partnerships. If digital technology is to play an active role in user participation in services, the latter must meet

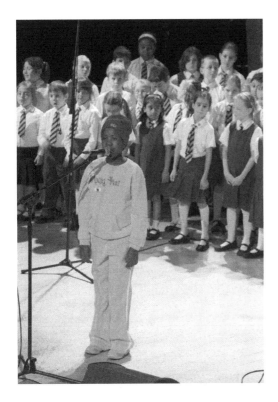

FIGURE 14 Brilliant Sango from Island Hospice, Zimbabwe performing with a choir from St Gabriel's Primary School, London at the songrooms launch concert at The Unicorn Theatre, London, December 2006.

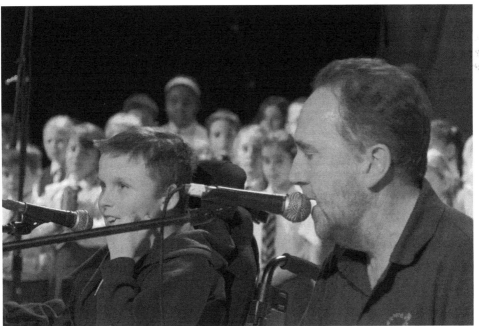

FIGURE 15 Daniel Dean and his carer, Bernie Wrighton from Richard House Children's Hospice, London performing their song at the songrooms launch concert at The Unicorn Theatre, December 2006.

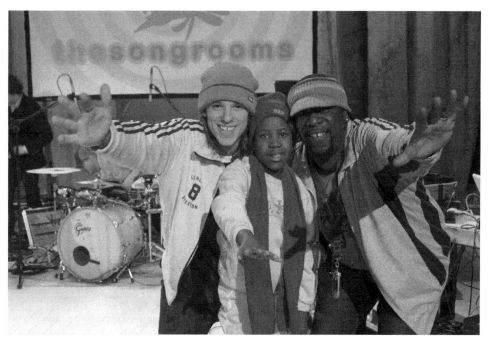

FIGURE 16 The songrooms launch concert at The Unicorn Theatre, December 2006. (From left) Theo Gordon, Brilliant Sango, Ricky Rankin.

a number of prior requirements. E-services must be available to palliative care users, supported by training and well-resourced and affordable systems.

If we introduce digital technology as a principle of driving user involvement in care, then we could witness the revolution in healthcare that has affected the music and other media industries. Dr Jeremy Keen, consultant in palliative care at Highland Hospice is keen to provide online access for patients and suggests that one way to make patient notes transparent and accessible might be to place them online and enable patients to update their own notes. Individual case notes become the kind of organic work in progress identified by James Walley, founder of Wikipedia.

The same open access could transform public education campaigns about death and dying. Last year Intel ran a campaign called 'Multiply Yourself' that enabled people to upload their picture onto a 19 200 square foot billboard in Times Square. With corporate sponsorship the international hospice movement could easily duplicate this campaign and enable user's stories, poems and thoughts to be constantly uploaded to changing billboards in public places. In this way the hospice movement could deliver a public programme of social change that enables the dying to teach the living how to live.

Paul Laking, to whom this book is dedicated, texted me on New Year's Eve 2005, eight days before he died saying,

> 'The sky has never looked so beautiful. Suffolk beach. Best fireworks I have ever witnessed. Life has never been this brilliant.'

Through his mobile phone he shared his intense love of life with his friends before he died.

Allegedly, his last words were,

'I am about to find out what happens. I will know before you!'

This spirit of risk and adventure is at the heart of the journey faced by those who are using palliative care services. Let us embrace the adventure!

PART 4: MODELS OF GOOD PRACTICE FROM DIRECT EXPERIENCE

CHAPTER 15

Poems for World Day

Lucinda Jarrett

Message from Nick Pahl

Help the Hospices facilitated the first World Hospice and Palliative Care Day in 2005 because we wanted to connect with as many people as possible about care at the end of life, how such care can help people and how much more needs to be done. I was amazed by the public's response – there were over 1100 events in 75 countries.

The theme in 2006 was 'access to care for all'. Hospice and palliative care services need to meet the challenge of how to widen access to all – for example to all disease groups, and not just for those with cancer. The commissioning of a Poems for World Day project occurred as a way of hearing from a new audience as part of this theme

Over the past few months I have been reading poems sent from all over the UK and around the world. I've been delighted by their humour, inspired by the profound depth of lives' explored, and been left humbled by brutal honesty.

Thanks to everyone involved.

Nick Pahl
International Development Director, Help the Hospices

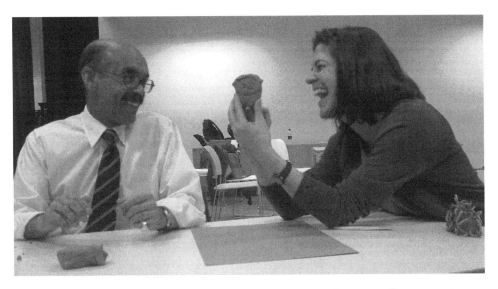

FIGURE 17 Poetry workshop at Tate Modern, August 2006 with Eddie Gittens (hospice service user) and Mariana Giovino (volunteer) from Trinity Hospice.

Introduction

Lucinda Jarrett

When Nick Pahl invited us to design a project for World Hospice and Palliative Care Day we worked hard to come up with one that would enable the palliative care community to participate fully and make their voice heard. Poems for World Day is a poetry project that enabled people working within or using palliative care to express their thoughts and feelings online. To kickstart the project, we invited leading poets to help people get involved. Wendy Cope set out some guidelines for writing poetry to get people started (see below), and Adrian Mitchell gave us permission to reprint his poem, 'Twenty One Secrets of Poetry', which was particularly targeted at children. Throughout the summer poets ran workshops across the country – Alice Oswald worked at Leckhampton Court Hospice in Gloucestershire (see interview with her below) and Zenobia Venner worked at Trimar Hospice in Weymouth. Roger Robinson donated CDs and books of his poems to inspire children in hospices and Rosetta Life ran workshops at the Tate Modern. Francesca Beard joined the judging panel and Patience Agbabi kindly agreed to MC the Poems for World Day awards at Tate Modern on 6 October.

When the judging panel met to shortlist the finalists we were looking for poems that demonstrated clarity of voice, writers with strong identities and stories that felt authentic. We also wanted a selection of poems that included the international context of palliative care and the diversity of this global community.

The poems people submitted are about relationships past and present, the hospices where they received care and the experiences of life and illness. We were deeply moved and impressed by the honesty of the writing, the humour, love and understanding of the emotions expressed, and the strength of the human spirit in the face of difficulty, illness and pain.

I am particularly pleased that the individual voice can be heard so clearly in this anthology. The rise of performance poetry in our culture – that emphasises the spoken rather than the written word – has been a boost to creative writing in hospices because it has enabled people to focus on their own voice and the stories they have to tell, instead of poetic techniques of metre and rhythm. What shines out from this project is how many hospice staff and service users have found a creative voice to celebrate life even in the middle of illness and death.

Keeping an open mind

Andy Fagg

An interview with Alice Oswald

When Alice Oswald told people that she was collaborating with hospice users she got a typical reaction. Eyes became sad and people commented, 'It must be difficult'. Her actual experience, at Leckhampton Hospice in Gloucestershire, was quite the opposite and can be symbolised by the difficulty she had in hearing the recordings she made in the hospice.

'There is a happy atmosphere in the hospice,' she said. 'When I listened back to some of the tapes I couldn't hear some words for the laughter and hubbub in the background. It's not what people expect a hospice to be like.'

Her poetry workshops at Leckhampton began during the summer. In the first, she spoke generally about poetry, read some of her own poems and asked those attending to write about a communal experience. Several hospice users were instantly captivated. Working in a small group, they engaged in fevered discussions about contemporary poetry. Alice's challenge was to redefine poetic form in a way that satisfied them. In every meeting they talked about what made poetry when structure was taken away. Gradually, the group were liberated from preconceived ideas about what poetry should be and began to write much more interestingly about their experiences.

Working in a small group passionate about discovering poetry was fine, but Alice quickly became uncomfortable working with large groups. She said: 'A lot of people were hostile to the idea of writing. People have a difficulty with poetry – perhaps as a hangover from how it was taught at school. So the challenge was to put across that it is about exploring experiences rather than following a regimented set of literary rules.'

Alice was challenged by an expectation that she was there to provide 'tricks' for writing poems. For a poet who finds writing a slow process – 'each time I write a poem I go through weeks with my head in my hands. It takes me to such an intense place' – the only realistic way to move ahead was to collaborate on a one-to-one basis.

For her 2002 award-winning poem, 'Dart', about people who live and work on the River Dart in her Devon homeland, she spent two years assembling a 'sound map' to capture accurately their unique voices and characteristics. She employed the same technique in collaboration with the hospice users, taping them in interviews that would typically last an hour. She asked them to talk about their interests. The length of the interview meant that however reluctant or unsure the hospice user was, by the time an hour was up a central experience or narrative had emerged.

Alice transcribed the recordings at home and took them back to the hospice for discussion. Working with sound proved successful. 'People naturally speak poetry. When they turn to paper, they turn it into something literary,' she said.

Though the hospice users explored a wide range of subjects, trends and common experiences surfaced. Women, for instance, were freer when talking about domestic life and men about their achievements and their work. World War II, its hardships and struggle, came up frequently. Alice said that people used their experiences and memories of the war as a way of gauging and articulating their amazement at how much the world had changed since. Mothers, too, were regularly talked about.

Alice said: 'I saw what an effect people's mothers had on them. They still dwelt on things their mother said to them. As a mother myself, it was fascinating to see that the influence was so strong.'

Fellow writer Jeanette Winterson has called Alice Oswald 'a Nature poet, a spiritual poet'. Did this help when she came to collaborating with people who might be dying? She said: 'Writing about nature is all about keeping an open mind and keeping your senses absolutely open so you are not projecting your image on the world. I tried to do the same during the interviewing: be completely open to who they are and just listen.'

In this attempt at an authentic realisation of individual experience she said she learned more than she was able to impart. 'I feel I've been given a completely new perspective: to see my own life much more in its wholeness. It's wonderful to speak to people who feel they are at the end of their lives – to see people who are just themselves. I wouldn't have missed these sessions for anything,' she said.

Some thoughts and suggestions about writing poems

Wendy Cope

Beginning

In the early 1970s I read an essay by RD Laing called 'The Politics of Experience'. At one point he writes about drawing a pattern on a piece of paper. 'Am I amazed', he asks, 'that something has appeared that did not exist before? That these lines did not exist on this paper until I put them there? Here we are approaching the *experience of creation* ...'

In the following paragraph he says this about the creation of a poem: 'Through all the contention of intention and motives a miracle has occurred. There is something new under the sun; being has emerged from nonbeing; a spring has bubbled out of a rock.'

Those two paragraphs liberated me. I understood that I was free to make any mark I liked on a piece of paper. I began to write poems.

At first it was a private and secret activity. I needed to remind myself that I didn't have to show my poems to anybody, or submit them to any judgement but my own. I certainly wasn't thinking of trying to get them published. I was enjoying myself, playing with words, trying to craft them into accurate accounts of my experience. I look back on this time with some nostalgia, as an age of innocence before I began worrying about editors, critics, or the reading public. Ever since I have known that to produce anything good, I have to find my way back into that state of mind, where I write what the hell I want to write and don't worry about what anyone else is going to think.

At the same time I began reading a lot of poetry – recent poetry, and the poetry of past centuries. I could see that the poems I was reading were much better than my own, and I learned from them. That's how a person learns to write poems: by reading poems. I found there were certain poets whose work I especially liked. Many of my early poems, I now see, are poor imitations of these poets. That's a phase that most of us have to go through, and we learn from it.

Of course, everyone is free to write whatever he or she likes, and there's no law that says you have to read other people's work, or learn anything about technique. But if you happen to believe that anything worth doing is worth doing well, you will want to work at it.

Working at it

It is very unusual for a person's first attempt at writing a poem to be entirely successful, although it may show promise. I have known brilliant people who couldn't write at all because they could tell that their initial efforts weren't very good, and they lacked the humility to write the bad stuff, and then work at it. That's what we all have to do, if we want to write good poems.

As I said above, reading poems is by far the most important thing. But books about writing poetry can also be stimulating and useful. There are books that will help you understand metre and traditional forms, and that give advice on writing well in free verse.

Some insecure people use a special voice on the telephone that sounds quite different from the way they usually speak. Inexperienced writers sometimes do something similar in their poems – using 'poetic' language that would never employ in ordinary speech. Stick to the language of ordinary speech. Ask yourself 'Would I use this word if I were talking to somebody?' The aim is to find your own voice. Since each of us is a unique individual, that voice will be unique. The real voice of a real person is one of the elements that make a poem readable.

A good question to ask yourself, if a poem isn't working, is 'Am I telling the truth?' TS Eliot said that the greatest difficulty for a poet is to distinguish between 'what one really feels and what one would like to feel'. You need to search for the words and images that accurately convey the truth of the matter. This doesn't mean that everything in a poem has to be literally true – I'm talking about truth to feeling.

- Show, don't tell. This advice is reiterated on hundreds of creative writing courses. An example of telling: 'she was upset'; of showing: 'she sniffed and reached for a tissue.'
- Notice details and choose carefully which ones to put in your poem. One good detail can say more than a whole gang of abstract nouns.
- When you are working on a poem, keep all the drafts. You may want to go back to an earlier version. I work in a large hardback notebook, so nothing gets lost.
- I also have a little notebook that goes in my handbag. But the back of an envelope will do. Poetry is a wonderfully portable art-form. Just make sure you always have a biro or a pencil on you.

Sharing your poems

Although privacy and secrecy were important at first, I reached a point where I needed to share my poems with other people and get some feedback. I had a colleague at work who wrote poems. When I mentioned that I'd been writing some, he insisted on seeing them. I was extremely nervous as I sat there watching him read my poems. Fortunately for me, he was very encouraging. After that I branched out, going on courses and becoming part of a workshop group.

The following information may be of use:

- the Poetry Society (020 7420 9880 or info@poetrysociety.org.uk) runs a service called Stanza, which helps people get in touch with others who want to be part of a poetry group
- the same society offers a Prescription Service. In return for a fee you can send in a specified number of poems for constructive criticism by a published poet. (Please don't send unsolicited work to published poets, expecting them to provide this service.)
- the literature officer at your regional arts association may know of workshop groups in your area
- the Arvon Foundation offers five-day courses on writing poetry and on other kinds of writing. The tutors are published writers, and the maximum number of students is around 16. There are Arvon centres in Devon, Yorkshire, Shropshire and Scotland. Bursaries are available for people who can't afford the fee. I attended several of these courses and found them very helpful. If you're wondering if you are well enough to go on a course, it might be a good idea to have a chat with the centre manager before booking. Details are available on the Arvon Foundation website or contact the Arvon national office at 42a Buckingham Palace Road, London SW1W 0RE
- Ty Newydd, the creative writing centre in North Wales, is not part of the Arvon Foundation but it is run on the same lines. Telephone 01766 522811 or email post@tynewydd.org.

Publication

Many people who write poems feel that their efforts are wasted unless they get published. This is a shame. Think of all the amateur musicians and amateur painters whose lives are enriched by their artistic work, although they don't get invited to give concerts on the South Bank or exhibit their work in a major gallery. They may well be enriching the lives of their friends and families as well.

You can share a poem with one person, or a group of people. These days it is very easy to print off multiple copies of a poem, or to email it to a number of people. In the years to come, your poems may be very precious to your loved ones.

I once stayed with a farming family in Yorkshire who showed me a book of poems by a late uncle. They had arranged for the book to be printed and given to him on his 80th birthday. It must have meant a lot to him, and the poems still, evidently, meant a lot to them.

If you want to try and publish for a wider audience, the first step is usually to try poetry magazines. A list of these, and of publishers of poetry books, is available on the website of the Poetry Library. The library itself, situated in the Royal Festival Hall, is closed for renovation until June 2007. For further information I recommend *How To Publish Your Poetry* by Peter Finch (published by Allison and Busby).

Wendy Cope is a Fellow of the Royal Society of Literature and lives in Winchester.

Below are the shortlisted poems selected from the online submissions. The poems were selected by a panel of judges that comprised performance poet Francesca Beard; David Hart, chair of Help the Hospices Users Group; Lucinda Jarrett; Nick Pahl, International Development Manager, Help the Hospices.

The Olive Tree
Jim McCleod
Greenwich and Bexley Cottage Hospice, UK

Six weeks ago I should have died
And didn't
My feet swelled up
This arm was thicker than that leg
I should've died but didn't
This week I walked across the room without a frame
I felt revitalised
Last night I lay awake, moving my fingers
And it felt good
In Greece, when the olive tree won't fruit
They wrap it in mattresses and sacking
Then bash it, knock it about generally
They stimulate a storm
The tree is revitalised
Invigorated
And fruits again

Jim McCleod, a Scot who lived in England for many years, loved observing nature. Looking out of the window from his bed in Greenwich and Bexley Cottage Hospice he noticed something amiss with the seasons – hedgehogs hibernating too early, oak trees budding twice, foxes with second litters in one year. 'Out of balance,' is what he called it. He could see the effects of global warming all around him. Jim died 10 July 2006.

Woof!
Josh Smith
Richard House Hospice, UK

My puppy is brown
And small
And very friendly

Woof! Woof! Woof! Woof!
Woof! Woof! Woof! Woof!

He's soft
And cuddly
And has many playful puppy friends.

Woof! Woof! Woof! Woof!
Woof! Woof! Woof! Woof!

I've had him since I was two
He makes me feel happy.
And he's very, very clever -
He can count up to eight.

Woof! Woof! Woof! Woof!
Woof! Woof! Woof! Woof!

Josh is an 8-year-old boy who is chatty, creative and imaginative. At Richard House Children's Hospice he likes to get involved in really fun stuff like Ghost Hunts, making up plays and playing with Scalextrix sets. Josh wrote this poem about his toy dog 'Puppy' who is very special to him and has been his trusted companion for much of his life.

Fred is Dead
Sue Lattey
Phyllis Tuckwell Hospice, UK

I'm sorry to hear that Fred has gone.
Gone where?
What do they mean?
Has he gone for a walk, gone abroad,
to do the shopping or to the pub?
Why can't they say that Fred is dead?

What! Fred's passed over?
Passed over what?
Passed over the road or the river?
He could never run, so it's not the baton in a relay race.
What they mean is
Fred is dead.

I regret that Fred has passed on.
I know that Fred has passed on so much to me.
I have the house, the car, the debts are all paid.
Fred taught me to mend a fuse,
to change a plug, to change a wheel and maintain the car
Why regret that?
No I'm pleased.
What I regret is
Fred is dead.

I'm sorry to hear that Fred is dead.
You will miss him.
At last in those few words,
probably felt to be inadequate,
someone knows how I feel.
I will miss him, his humour,
his company, the early morning tea,
the shared views, the love of cats,
the annoying cough, the toothpaste tube!
Nevertheless that was love.
Moreover I have my memories.
No one can take that away.
With that understanding from this true friend
I can get on with my life.
Now I can say –
Fred is dead, long live Fred.

Sue has been working as a nurse at the Phyllis Tuckwell Hospice in Farnham for 16 years. While studying palliative care she wrote this poem. She said: 'I feel that the use of euphemisms can prevent some people from facing and accepting the death of a loved one. This in turn can delay the grieving process. Where friends feel unable to mention the words, "death" and "dead", the bereaved person can find it much harder being true to their feelings in the company of these people.' Married to Peter, with two children, Sue is also an unpaid priest at the parish church in Ash Vale.

escalier
Astrid Guillermin
Centre de Soins Palliatifs Lyon Sud, France

Comme il descend vite l'escalier en spirale.
Tout est rond, interminable, entêtant.
Dans ses bras, des feuilles et des cahiers
Chargés de contes, de maximes et de poèmes

A chaque marche descendue, une feuille s'enfuit, s'envole

Que faire de ce trésor lorsque la symphonie stridente et
Sombre à la fois, grise et cruelle, déchire murs et jardins
Comme du carton?

L'escalier tourne encore et toujours et l'homme court
Bientôt la fin; voici l'abri.
Il ne reste à l'homme qu'un seul poème qu'il pose sur la table.

Poème d'amour luttant de tous ces fruits contre l'entourage maudit
de la poussière et des coups.

Puis les familles arrivent dans la nuit, en quête de sécurité.
Elles lisent le poème et le murmurent.
Et les mots d'amour, petit à petit, éteignent la symphonie maudite
Et demain existe, ce soir.

Il y aura un nouveau destin.

staircase
Translation by Lucinda Jarrett

Look how quickly he runs down the spiral staircase.
Everything circles round, dizzying, endless.
In his arms his pages and notebooks
Are full of stories, ideas and poems

As he descends each step, a page flees, takes flight

What should he do with this treasure, now that this symphony at once screeching
And somber, grey and cruel, is tearing at the walls and the gardens
As if they were cardboard?

The staircase turns again and still the man is running down
Almost there now: here is the shade.
He has only one poem left and he places it on the table.

It is a love poem that is fighting in all its incarnations against
The cursed surroundings and the dust and the bullets.

Now the families arrive in search of safety as it gets dark.
They read the poem and whisper it.
And the words of love, little by little extinguish the cursed symphony.
And this evening, tomorrow exists.

There will be a new future.

Astrid was a tour guide and interpreter based in Lyon, where she was born in 1959. She was highly influenced by a visit to Lebanon in 1999, writing travel diaries and a collection of poems about the country. She was gravely affected by the recent war in Lebanon and wrote 'escalier' on her hospital bed – her last homage to a country she loved. She died from cancer on 28 August 2006, leaving her husband, Frederick, and their two little girls, Sophie and Lucy.

I Watched You as You Died

Kogi Singh
Chatsworth Regional Hospice Association, South Africa

I watched you as you died, Mother -
my Ma, suddenly re-Christened *Marmie* in our pretentious teenage years.
How you laughed then, your fancy caught by your love
of wailing bagpipes and your new Scottish-inspired name!

Mother. A single word that defies an all-encompassing meaning,
that cannot describe the softness, the warmth, the smiling eyes and
open arms. The essential you.

I heard your struggle to breathe, the harsh, raucous sound
an abrasive intrusion into the stillness that surrounded us,
that held us unmoving, whispering, as though we might disturb you.
But you had already gone far away.

I held your hand, stroked softly through your thinning grey hair
unable to ease your pain, remembering other times
when you held me close, bathed my fevered cheeks and crooned softly
- mesmeric, comforting, a soothing vibration
like the heartbeat that thrummed through me as I nestled
in your womb.

I prayed you would open your eyes, see me before you go
let me show you how much I love you.
But you lay there, locked in stasis, no return pressure to hands
that held on to you, unwilling to let you go.
Only the stertorous, laboured breathing told us you were still there.

And then, shockingly, silence.
You opened your eyes, turned your head, looked at
the photograph of Papa on the wall beside you
and died.

I understand now how much you wanted to go.
It has helped to bring a quiet acceptance and even joy.
Be happy, Mother, and thank you.

Kogi is a South African woman, a retired educator aged 67, married to a fellow educator. She has written a biography entitled *A Labour of Love* (2000) about a local man who dedicated his entire life to the service of the poor, the needy and the sick. Her interest has now moved to poetry and short story writing. Her three children and five grandchildren all live in Durban, which she said makes her life happily hectic. She serves as a volunteer for Chatsworth Regional Hospice Association in Durban.

Approximately 10 Things Which are Wonderful, in No Order
Nancy Jeanie Brown
Hospice in the Weald, UK

Deep warm bubble bath with candles & incense, watching the fish as I soak. Real fires: inside & outside giving warmth to all senses. Waking up with Andy next to me, reminding me every morning of what love feels like. The first fall of fresh snow, and the feeling of 'cold' on your face. Having MacDuff: a place in my heart is just for him. Long chats & laughs & going shopping with friends. The moments you have when you read a passage in the Bible, and you feel God talking to you. Going back to bed after breakfast, because you can. Listening to tunes in the car, with the roof down. Watching nature unfold, Everywhere.
Swimming in the sea.

Reliving memories in your mind...

These are some of the things wonderful to me.

Nancy was born and brought up in Glasgow. She studied textile design at the Scottish College of Textiles, majoring in weave. After graduation in 1989 she moved to Manchester to design fabrics in different technologies for the automotive market. She travelled to all of the major car manufacturers in Europe, Japan, China, Korea and North America. Later she managed the colour and materials team for Ford of Europe in London and Cologne. Since being diagnosed with breast cancer in October 2003 she has been living a 'very different, but far more rewarding life', having found more time to develop her creative skills in a personal way. She lives with husband Andy and cat 'Guzzi' in Sevenoaks, Kent.

Unwanted Guests
Beverly Ashill
Trinity Hospice, UK

An unwanted purple guest came to my house one night –
She has been there ever since.
How she got in I do not know,
For I was sure my doors were locked.
But there she was, inside me
Vibrant and bold and purple,
Unafraid she made me scared.
I have tried to poison her many times.
Sometimes the poison makes her sleep for a time,
But then she wakes,
Angry and vengeful,
She rapes me repeatedly
Behind closed bedroom doors.
Having no voice of her own
She steals mine, rendering me silent.
Not content with her own company,
She brought a friend –
A chunky blue snake who wrapped herself around me crushing my breath
The snake had babies: I was her womb.
They are my family now:
Should they leave one night,
Slamming the door behind them,
Would I be lost?

Beverley Ashill is a singer and actor who recently lost her voice due to cancer. Although she is still hoping to recover her voice, writing is giving her a new means of creative expression. Her first serious attempt at writing was for Rosetta Life's online song-cycle project 'Rosetta Requiem'. Her lyrics were used by classical composer David Matthews to create a piece for soprano and strings.

Simpson's Gap, Northern Australia

Pat Goodhew
Leckhampton Court Hospice, UK

Today a butterfly drank from my hand.
A coach stop at Simpson's Gap
In the dry-tongued brittle heat of the Red Heart.
'Go and see the rock wallabies' said our guide,
'but keep together, go quietly and don't forget to drink.'
Whooping and shouting they piled out.......
'Quick, quick, let's see how far we can go.'
'Run, run. I can go further than you.'
Left behind, I turned from the track and sat on a log
And as the torn silence settled down again
I heard the tick-tock sound of the bush.
Then, remembering, drank from my water bottle,
A few drops falling sparkling on my hand.
At once, down came a bright beauty.
Landed on my hand – I felt the flicker of its feet.
It drank, quivering, until the drops were gone.
Then it fluttered the fan of its wings
And then was away, that bright beauty.
I felt the air softly stir on my finger
As the bush settled around me again.
I did not see the rock wallabies
But a butterfly drank from my hand today.

Brought up on the edge of Epping Forest near the North Weald aerodrome, Pat had a good view of the Battle of Britain. Perhaps it was seeing the planes that gave her a thirst for travel. After the war, she trained as a primary school teacher and later married an Australian-born naval officer while teaching in Malta. She visited Australia around 15 years ago and had the trip of her life. It included the intimate moment described in this poem.

Feelings
Collette Waller
Greenwich and Bexley Cottage Hospice, UK

The other day, well
Three in the morning it was
I said to my Dad
Who was awake
I feel so depressed
He paused, then said
Don't use that word
You're not
I said, alright then I'm frustrated

The Traveller
Collette Waller
Greenwich and Bexley Cottage Hospice, UK

I'd like to say
I've been here and done this
Been there and done that
The fact is I ain't been nowhere
Recently

Collette Waller has progressive secondary Multiple Sclerosis. Before her diagnosis, she was communication manager for the Daily Telegraph and played netball for Kent and Surrey. She has been collaborating with Rosetta Life artist Chris Rawlence for the last few years at Greenwich and Bexley Cottage Hospice to write poetry, much of which has provided lyrics for her character in the Rosetta Life musical, *The Mariners*.

The Tear and The Telescope
Kate Woodman
Hospice in the Weald, UK

The tear said to the telescope
'People see more through me'
The telescope replied
'Oh really, how can that be?'
'They see deep down into my soul'
The tiny tear replied
'I show sorrow, grief and scars
While you see only distant stars'
'But I can magnify the world'
The telescope replied
'You are just a drop of dew
In someone's crying eyes'
'I don't agree', the tear retorted
'I can help to get things sorted
Open floodgates of disaster
Or run with joy and fun and laughter'
'But I can see a million stars
And planets - Venus, Saturn, Mars
I can cross the seven seas
So I'm the greatest, if you please!'
'But I am precious to the world,'
The tiny tear went on
'I show compassion, grief and pain
Helping people take the strain
Of all the things they have to bear
While all you do is stand and stare'
'Alright', the telescope conceded
'I guess you're right
But tell your eyes
When tears have dried
That I can help to open wide
A world of joy in secret skies
Hidden from the naked eyes
So let's agree to work together
You show joy and pain and pleasure
While I show galaxies and treasure'
'Oh, yes!' the tear replied
'I see your point,
We both are blessed by God above
Who sends us different gifts of love'
And so the two walked hand in hand
Throughout the world
As God had planned.

Kate Woodman attends the Hospice in the Weald in Sussex. She is a dancer and a poet who is inspired by her Christian faith.

Barbie Princesses hee hee hee
Olivia Inns and Jo
Richard House Hospice, UK

Jo, Olivia's nurse:

I've known Olivia for five years now
She loves the nail varnish on her toes

And likes the mirrors so she can watch herself play
Makes sure she looks pretty all day

She loves hearing her toy turn round and round
The mirrors and bells make a lovely sound.

A Disney wand rings out princess voices
Like her, beautiful in pink enjoying the noises.

Olivia:

Hello. I'm Cinderella
Let's make our dreams come true.

Nk. Gnk. Gnk. Gn. Gnk.

I'm Snow White.
How do you do?

Wfffh Wfffh Wfffh
Cool air on our cheeks

GNk. GGNK. k. nk. Gn. Gnk.
Vib-rat-ing gums.

Touch of teeth on teeth
Jaw. Gnaw. Gn. Jaw

Stampf Mmmppf mmpf
Feet on soft sheet.

Hello. I'm Belle.
Are you ready for magic?

Toes become fingers
Holding the toy
Tongue licking the base
Sensing wood on tongue
Fingering toes turn the bells

Ink clink. Clin. In. k.k.
Ack.Clack.cllck.cllck.

Mirr-or-ing clinking belling
Turning tirning clinking singing

Hee hee heee. Giggl-e –e -hee-

Hello I'm Cinderella
Let's wave the magic wand.

Wfffh Wfffh Wfffh

Stampf Mmmppf mmpf Ink clink. Clin. In. k.k.Ack.Clack.cllck.cllck.

Stampf Mmmppf mmpf GNk.

GGNK. k. nk. Gn. Gnk.

Ink clink. Clin. In. k.k.

Hee hee heee.

Olivia is a very pretty seven-year-old girl who has the most contagious giggle and always dresses in very trendy clothes. She likes playing with musical and girly toys and looking at all the amazing lights in the multi-sensory room at Richard House. Olivia cannot verbally communicate, so instead she lets everyone know what she wants and how she is feeling by using her voice and her facial expressions.

My Darkest Night
Helen Sanford
North Shore Hospice, New Zealand

In the deepest sleep of my darkest night
The dream of the Golden Butterfly came to me
She showed me passages of my life, in images
First born, an egg – pearly white – perfect

When the time was perfect, the caterpillar emerged
Searching for sustenance, needing, urging to grow
As she grew bigger so her life grew shorter, shorter
When she could be no more, she died to the chrysalis

And the Dream Maker spoke her wisdom to me...
'That part of your life is gone, yes
And a new one about to begin
You must struggle in your release
And you must be on your own
As you cast off the shell of the old life
Your inner beauty as a butterfly will unfold
So as you transform, a new life will be
To be again, totally perfect and complete
And as before, your love and passion
Will radiate over others and you will give again
And you will never be forgotten, never'

Sunrise woke me from the sleep of my darkest night
Had I dreamed a butterfly taught me of life and death
That when I die my body will fall away as a cocoon
And my life will go on, that I will forever be ...... LOVE

Helen writes: 'I am a mother of three awesome adult children and am constantly inspired by many aspects of their natures but their love and ability to forgive touches my heart most. Next to my children, my life's work is as a hospice nurse, a privilege I have been blessed with for the last seven years. In my life there have been many influences which have brought me to where I am today, none less or more significant than the other. Every moment of extreme hardship, blessed bliss and what was in between has taught me something about what love is and for these gifts I am truly grateful.

Ah Bless
Mary Winton
Trimar Hospice, UK

She's not been well
Ah bless

Proper poorly she's been
Ah bless

Had Breast Cancer, she did
Ah bless

And chemotherapy too
Ah bless

It took six months to sort
Ah bless

She had some good support
Ah bless

Her family and friends did help
Ah bless

She's all better now
Ah bless

Got a new job now as well
Ah bless

Has got the all clear
Ah bless

Time to move on
Ah bless

Mary decided she wanted to write poems when she was standing at her kitchen sink and saw a flock of migrating geese fly overhead. She said it has been good to let off some steam. 'I wanted to write about the different ways of saying "Ah bless",' she said. 'Sometimes it can be very sad, but other times it can be patronising.' Mary lives with her father, three cats and a dog and works as an assistant in a shoe shop.

Meriel
Frank Hill
St Barnabas Hospice, UK

Meriel,
It's just a name,
A single word,
Yet whisper it and then for me that simple single world becomes,
A symphony.

Frank writes: 'I am a 70-year-old man with an incurable bone marrow shut down called Aplastic Anemia. Enough of that, I attend St Barnabas House twice a week giving respite to both my wife (truly beloved) and myself, stimulating both our brains in different directions.'

Palliative Care
Job Wekesa Wamukaya
Kenya

Thanks to Palliative care approach
The approach has no comparison
Palliative care transforms life
It gives hope to the hopeless
Palliative care is a 'U' TURN
It is a source and a well of springs of Hope

Palliative care has improved quality of life
It is a granary to reap from
Palliative care relieves suffering
Pain is managed to nothing by Palliative treatment
It provides walking aids, wheel chairs and beds
It is a source and a well of springs of hope.

Palliative care for those diagnosed terminally ill
Life is threatened by the illness to no where to turn to
Palliative care team has opened hands to receive you.
No visitor comes to your doorstep, no friend
Nor relative knocks your door
Palliative care team pays you a visit
It is a source and a well of springs of hope.

Palliative care makes symptoms meaningless
Vomiting, diarrhea, itching skin, constipation
Physical, psychological, spiritual problems
Palliative care controls them all, it is an answer
It is a source and a well of springs of hope.

Palliative care a wonderful approach
If I were a musician I could compose you a song
Palliative care is like salt for food, it tastes
It is a lit lamp in the darkness of terminal illness
A forest of problems in terminal illness
Palliative care is a path through that forest
It is a source and a well of springs of hope.

Palliative care in bereavement
Dying is borne normally.
The bereaved have support to cope
It offers this indiscriminately,
Readily available and timely support
Just like breast milk
It is a source and a well of springs of hope.

My Boat
Rosalyn Newman
Lion's Hospice, UK

I like fish,
I like boats,
I like to go in the middle of the ocean:
My boat is green; I am a yellow figure;
My big friendly fish swims under me,
Green eyes, the only fish with green eyes.
I would like to be there on my boat:
Problem is, my husband doesn't come with me.
He doesn't like boats.

Rosalyn lived in Zamboanga City in the Philippines until 1986 when she came to Kent working as a psychiatric nursing assistant at Joyce Green Hospital, Dartford. It was whilst she was at the hospital that she met her husband to be, Trevor. Rosalyn has always been interested in writing poetry and despite having to overcome the difficulty of coping with a strange new language, is able to express herself beautifully in verse.

The Spider Inside
Dorothy Trewartha
Trimar, UK

She's lurked in my body
For too many years
Growing bigger and scarier
Just like my fears

She sits in a corner
And sends out her thread
To my back, to my lung,
To my liver, (my head?)

'Why should it be me?'
'Why not?' she replies,
'Someone else didn't get it
and everyone dies.'

'You have many blessings
and faced up to your fear
I'm a **very** slow grower
which is why you're still here.'

Dorothy was born and brought up in the shipbuilding northwest coastal town of Barrow-in-Furness. A Trimar day patient in Dorset, she has fought cancer for more than 20 years. In this poem she suggests that her many blessings and her ability to face up to fears have meant the spider, a symbol of cancer, has grown slowly. She counts painting, writing, sitting in the garden, being by the coast and spending time with her family, including her much-loved grandchildren, among her many pleasures.

CHAPTER 16

Case study of service user forums at Dove House Hospice

Judith Hodgson

Getting beyond gratitude – service user forum experience at Dove House Hospice, Hull

Dove House is a hospice in Hull, a city in the north of England. It is a well established hospice and this year celebrates 25 years of offering specialist palliative care to the people of Hull and East Yorkshire. What started all those years ago as just a doctor, a social worker, a community nurse and a part time administrator is now a huge concern employing 130 paid staff and approximately 500 volunteers.

Introduction

Hospices are generally nice places to be, from both an employee's point of view and, of course, the many patients and relatives and carers who come to make use of the services available to them. Dove House Hospice, which has been in its present location for over fifteen years, has staff that have been there since the beginning. The joke is that they arrived with the cement mixer and bricks and never left. By and large it is a happy place to work offering a huge amount of job satisfaction. Of course, as in any organisation there have been occasional problems over the years, but generally these have been overcome and the hospice has moved forward.

From a patient's point of view coming to Dove House is a 'luxurious experience'. The facilities are 'wonderful', the food is 'great', the nurses are 'very kind', the doctors are 'very clever' and that doesn't include all the other associated services that make the hospice experience a positive one. These types of thoughts are likely to be further embedded if the patient has had a previous bad NHS experience. But even if their previous experience of the healthcare systems has been good, patients and their carers are likely to be pleasantly surprised with what a hospice has to offer.

An anecdote from some years back, which may be apocryphal, had a male patient come in to the hospice and refuse to eat. This confused all staff because a lack of appetite had not been a presenting symptom. However, when discussing the issue with the patient he said that he had not eaten because the place was so lovely and he expected to face a bill at the end of his stay which he would not be able to afford. Once it was explained (again) to him that the services were free an amazed patient started to 'tuck in' to the lovely food available. But so amazed and so grateful was he that after that he would not have a word said against the hospice and was constantly singing our praises.

And this is the problem. Hospices can be too nice, so much so that they discourage criticism. My own particular concern is that they also discourage anger. The pastel colours and kind environments do not encourage a patient to be furious because their life is coming to an end. So on the one hand through initiatives such as Service User Forums we are asking for criticism and comments and suggestions to improve our services yet on the other we are not providing an environment conducive to this. How do we therefore get beyond gratitude?

Initial concerns about service user involvement

> User involvement in palliative care raised its own particular challenges. This is because of the often rapidly changing circumstances and life-threatening illnesses which pallia-tive care users face.
>
> National Council for Hospice and Specialist Palliative Care Services
> Briefing number 6, November 2000

The idea of setting up a service user group was not a recently conceived concept here at Dove House Hospice. 'Buzz Groups' had been part of the hospice's early history and in these early groups service users met to discuss the services they had received. But even in those early days there had been concerns about the ethics involved and these remained. For some time the Bereavement Team had discussed the possibility of asking bereaved clients to assess the service and always there has been reluctance in case any good that might have been achieved by our intervention might be undone. On the Bedded Unit questionnaires were sent out some time after interventions came to an end but they tended to be of a nature which emphasised the practical side of the services offered and were not thought to be as emotionally risky. This new venture was different. We would be asking patients to comment on our services during interventions, much earlier in their hospice journey, and not only that, we were asking service users to make suggestions as to how these services could be improved.

The question posed here is, 'Whose needs are being met?' Are we meeting service user needs? Do they want or need to be so involved in the day to day running of the hospice? After all, they are usually so grateful and complementary about the services offered so therefore aren't we adding burdens to those who are already over-burdened by a life-limit-ing illness or grief. We know our services are good, the NICE Guidance recommends the specialist palliative care services offered by hospices so perhaps a little 'laurel-resting' would not be out of the question. Or are we meeting our own needs in order to prove to the various external regulatory bodies that our services are not only excellent but they have identified and documented service user approval.

Our starting point had to be therefore to ask service users:

- Did they think a service user forum would be helpful?
- Would they like to be part of it?

If these questions were given the affirmative we would take it further and the first meeting would be set up to test the water. This posed further questions. Would affirmative answers be given because of the gratitude we were trying to get away from? Would service users fully understand the issues and effort involved or was this a paternalistic viewpoint.

Beginnings

The decision was made. Dove House Hospice would have a Service User Forum, with perhaps a more friendly title evolving over time. There is no need to reinvent the wheel so we set about to find out who had a Service User Forum and pick their brains. Luckily the hospice movement is quite generous and there seems to be little in the way of 'This is our idea – get off'. We spotted a day planned to discuss setting up Service User Forums at St Christopher's Hospice and three of us set off to find out – an educationalist, a nurse and a social worker.

A number of things stood out from that day:

▨ the more planning that went into the project, the more I's dotted and T's crossed, the better the outcome
▨ a failsafe transport system was needed to bring people in and to get them home safe
▨ a nurse should be present and a doctor should be available at all times in case of difficulties arising and the particular difficulties of the illnesses of those attending should be noted
▨ the service users were doing us a favour and 'special' refreshments should be served to emphasise this
▨ the session should not last too long with plenty of refreshment and toilet breaks
▨ we should be aware that the group would change over time – some service users might be too ill to come and some may even have died since the last meeting
▨ three or four times a year were recommended times, avoiding the holiday periods in July and August
▨ the sessions needed to be advertised well in advance

Most of the above suggestions were adopted but with some exceptions and changes suggested by the service users themselves.

Preparation for meeting 1 – 20 February 2004

This was the inaugural meeting – to discuss the whole issue of a service user forum with service users. Was it wanted? Would it help? Would they come to meetings? If the service users said 'Yes' that would make things a lot simpler and a lot of our ethical and paternalistic concerns would be reduced. But what if they said 'No'? It was decided that if service users were not enthusiastic about the idea it would nevertheless remain and opportunities would still be available, whether in the form of open meetings or otherwise, for service users to share their thoughts and opinions. After all, the nature of the group would be constantly changing as would their points of view. A 'No' need not be a permanent 'No'.

Fliers and invitations were produced and distributed. For the first meeting we decided to keep within hospice boundaries i.e. patients on the Bedded Unit and Day Hospice would be the target group.

Which room to use?

The choice of room was a problem. Any old meeting room would just not do. It had to be comfortable and spacious (for wheelchairs) and welcoming. Our most spacious room with a reasonable welcome but not very comfortable was upstairs. We have a chairlift but was this asking too much of those who were keen to attend? Were we once again being too paternalistic? This upstairs room was discounted because it was too far from the toilets and getting a number of individuals up and down would be a logistical nightmare.

Another choice was Day Hospice. It was perfect. It was spacious and welcoming and had vast numbers of comfortable and supporting chairs. Toilets were within easy reach, sorting out refreshments would be easier and there were great views out into the garden. But Day Hospice was in use from Monday to Friday. To cancel a Day Hospice day for the sake of the forum was hardly meeting service user needs. But we figured that most people would come if it was a weekday. Both service users (and staff) might be reluctant to give up a precious Saturday and also if it was a weekday we had a captive audience – people who were likely to be invited might be already here. So although we agreed that a weekday was the best choice of day we were not prepared to lose a Day Hospice day. Therefore Day Hospice was discounted too.

This left the sitting room on the Bedded Unit. It was very comfortable but not over-spacious, an army of wheelchairs might make things a bit squashed and there might be problems at refreshment time. Toilets were nearby and it had the additional advantage of having doctors and nurses within very easy reach. But the biggest problem was that it was on the Bedded Unit itself, a place where a number of service users may have had bad experiences and associations and where it might be difficult for bereaved service users to return to should they also be invited at a later date. Was this paternalism raising its ugly head once again?

After a lot of unexpected thought and deliberation, we opted for the sitting room on the Bedded Unit. This was to be a feature of Service User Forum issues; what seems to be the simplest of problems invariably is not.

The first meeting

The first meeting was attended by 20 service users and 7 staff – perhaps too many staff. The purpose of the forum was explained. It was pointed out at this very early stage that it was very much a service user group and that the organisation did not want to dictate but also that all suggestions would be responded to even if they could not be put into practice. It was important to make clear that some suggestions might not be possible because of organisational and statutory rules and regulations. However if we had to say 'No' to something it would be accompanied by an explanation.

The twenty service users were enthusiastic both about the forum taking place and were keen to make lots of suggestions and voice their opinions – even to the extent of keeping the name, 'Service User Forum'. Suggestions were mainly of a practical nature – this had been the experience at St Christopher's Hospice also. The following were some of the suggestions:

- a video/book exchange for patients
- an allotment for patients
- more trips out (organised by patients)
- better bigger and clearer staff name badges
- Sky TV
- a debating society
- more creative writing.

But the service users were also critical and quite outspoken:

- why had the statue of Buddha gone from the garden?
- sometimes the patients were called "them" – this was not nice
- the proposed idea of a gym for the hospice was a daft idea and a waste of time
- why couldn't they have more baths?

But also positive and affirming:

▨ an open day would enable the public to see the good work taking place
▨ the atmosphere in the hospice was always warm and welcoming.

All in all it was felt by all concerned and involved that the first and inaugural meeting of the Service User Forum had been a success and that it should continue. It would take place every two months, a compromise, as service users had wanted the sessions to be monthly, but after discussion it was agreed that this was too frequent. Furthermore it should take place on a different day of the week each time to allow different Day Hospice patients to come each time with transport laid on for those from different Day Hospice days but who wished to attend the forum also. We had permission to continue!

Follow up

With the go-ahead came a commitment for staff to consider the suggestion and ideas. There then evolved another meeting – the Service User Feedback meeting which would be attended by the Chief Executive, the Chair and members of staff who attended regularly. Surprisingly it was not agreed in the first instance that a nominated service user should attend the Feedback meeting. This came later. The Feedback meeting would take place about a month after every forum. Some research has highlighted concerns that sometimes these feedback meetings were not a 'good thing'. Their very existence, however long after the meeting takes place, indicates that answers are not available immediately and that service users have to wait. Sometimes this cannot be helped given the nature of the question but perhaps it needs to be remembered that palliative care patients do not always have the luxury of time.

Most of the suggestions from the first meeting were met with a positive reaction but some had to be tempered. As a specialist palliative care service we are moving away from the traditional day hospice ideology of social time and entertainment to one where therapy is the main theme in which social time and entertainment are included. Therefore trips out and shopping are not as high on the agenda as they might have been in previous years and as a specialist palliative care service the patients who come our way are often too poorly to want to go out. So although this did not receive an unequivocal 'No', it received a 'Yes, perhaps' with reservations.

Meeting 2 – 1 April 2004

At the time of the second meeting Day Hospice was preparing for refurbishment and all of the day care services were moving offsite whilst the changes took place. This was a good opportunity for the Day Hospice patients to ask questions, offer ideas and air their concerns about the forthcoming changes. This was not so good in that it further embedded the forum as a service for Day Hospice service users. Most of this second forum was taken up with Day Hospice issues but there was also feedback from the questions asked during the first meeting.

Meeting 3 – 26 May 2004

Our third meeting! This meeting was significant in that the decision was made by all concerned that as the forum was up and running there was no need for a member of staff in a decision making role to be there. A volunteer was asked to accept this responsibility. He would manage the process but not the content and he along with a member of the social work team, who had been involved from the very beginning, would become the lead non-service users present. This gave consistency and familiarity to the meetings as both the volunteer and the social worker were well known on Day Hospice. It also presented opportunities to the service users to be more contentious in their suggestions which might not have been possible with a member of the senior management team present. It was also felt by this point that the forum belonged to the Service Users.

The main concerns at this meeting were once again the proposed changes to Day Hospice. The biggest item reported back from the first meeting was that better and clearer and colour coded name badges were on there way. Thus service users were able to see something tangible resulting from their thoughts and ideas.

An interesting item from this meeting was that the service users were keen to tell the world about the hospice and wished to put service information in the Dove House shops. However research shows that shoppers in charity shops do not want to know about the charity itself – it puts them off coming in and spending money. This idea was rejected but it does indicate that despite our efforts we were still facing the gratitude issue.

Meeting 4 – 20 July 2004

Once again the main topic for discussion was Day Hospice, newly christened Day Therapy and which was now re-established back at the hospice after refurbishment. There were many comments made, both positive and negative. Even the change of name from Day Hospice to Day Therapy was a topic for lively discussion. Again the concerns were mainly of a practical nature, e.g. the new meals system needed extra work, and they were met with generally positive reactions in the feedback meeting.

A particular feature of this meeting was discussion about the Bedded Unit. This was shortly to be refurbished and the service users who were often also patients on the Bedded Unit were keen to put forward their ideas.

Perhaps it should be noted at this point that the Service User Forum might have been such a success because major things were happening at the hospice that would encourage discussion. If there had been less activity affecting the daily living conditions of all those coming into the hospice would the discussion have been so lively? Change usually prompts discussion and there was a lot of change taking place.

Also many of the Day Therapy patients had diagnoses of longstanding neurological conditions and had been part of the hospice fabric for years. They were comfortable with the staff and the organisation in general, they felt a part of it and their prognoses were sufficiently fluid for them to believe they had a part to play in the hospice's future.

Meetings and feedback meetings have continued on a bi-monthly basis since and word got around to other hospices about our Service User venture. The achievements of the Service User Forum during the first year are considerable and are as follows:

- bigger and clearer name badges for all
- suggestion box in Day Therapy
- a review of physiotherapy services has led to the recruitment of another full time physiotherapist
- a review of Day Therapy transport has resulted in the purchase of a new ambulance
- Day Therapy has a putting green
- Day Therapy has a user led discussion group
- fire procedures have been reviewed and changed

■ more 'disabled' parking
■ increased user involvement in Dove House publications such as the Annual Report and a video
■ increased involvement in service planning, e.g. music therapy and refurbishment.

Preparation for a Listening Day

Once again instead of making assumptions about what the service users were capable of we decided to ask them. A Listening Day was arranged and all client groups were invited. Once again the thought and opinions of service users would be sought so that we could tackle the issues from their point of view.

In hindsight, we did not allow sufficient time for the preparation of this day. Invitations were sent out with insufficient thought attached to the guest list. All groups were invited – from Day Therapy, from the Bedded Unit and from our bereaved clients out in the community. Unfortunately there was no cut off point for the bereaved clients and clients whose loss was some months in the past were invited alongside those whose losses had been more recent. Also some of the bereaved clients had issues with Dove House itself, some of these issues were real and some indicated the direction of their grief that would be resolved in time.

This posed lots of questions. Were we again being too paternalistic and over-protective? Wasn't the forum the perfect place for ALL issues?

The Listening Day itself

Feedback from the thirty service users who attended the day indicated that the Listening Day was a success. The day went as follows.

Arrival and refreshments

This was unintentionally staggered and because of transport problems some service users arrived after the beginning of our day together and we felt that they had difficulty in getting involved. This needs more thought next time and was, after all, one of the issues raised at St Christopher's at that very early meeting.

Generally this was a settling in period where the service users got to know each other, got to know the staff in whose group they would be and also where, as far as possible, newcomers to Dove House were helped to feel at home. For many it was home from home but for some it was the first visit altogether or the first visit after a death and it was important that their specific needs were met.

Group work

This was the formal part of the day and the service users were divided into mixed groups together with two members of staff to discuss services they had received and how they think they should be developed. In one group the combination was fine and the bereaved service users, patients and carers mixed very well with lively discussion and a healthy openness in the very different problems they were facing. In one group, however, the mix was not a success and a bereaved service user needed more support than had been anticipated and the group did not find it easy to be supportive. Rather the group process was disrupted by it.

In one of the groups the discussion got round to respite care. Or at least the discussion got round to how poor respite care facilities were in this area. The sad fact that younger patients with neurological conditions often had to go into nursing or residential accommodation for respite care where they might be surrounded by other residents twice their age was acknowledged but with regret. Even coming into Dove House Hospice for respite care was not always ideal as very often the carer came in every day early in the morning and stayed until the evening. My own casework history at Dove House Hospice includes a client whose husband suffered from multiple sclerosis and who came into Dove House for regular respite care or pain and symptom control. The carer/wife used every opportunity that her husband was in the hospice to decorate a room and usually when he returned home she was more tired than when he was admitted. Respite care does not always mean that the carer and patient needed to be separated. Perhaps they need to be together but away from all the rest of their care and responsibilities.

A result of this discussion, where the Chief Executive and Chair were present, was that the Board of Trustees should look once again at the idea that we have a family respite care centre built to meet such need. The Board did agree to this proposal and at the time of writing plans have gone ahead for a family respite care facility with full disabled facilities to be built on a small site in the grounds of a nearby stately home. This facility in the form of a wooden chalet will have two bedrooms and patients who are facing a life-limiting illness plus their families will be able to make use of it. Plans are still in the early stage.

We hope it will be used by patients both with cancer and those with a neurological condition. My own opinion is that it will be well used by patients with multiple sclerosis who cannot travel far. Some of our patients with multiple sclerosis would love to visit the multiple sclerosis centre at York, a mere 45 miles away, but the journey would be too much for them. This new facility is only a twenty minute car journey from the hospice and well within the range of most of our service users.

Lunch

This was a cooked lunch and not a cold buffet and was enjoyed by all. This was one lesson from St Christopher's that we had learned well – the refreshments need to be of a good quality. Lunch was very informal and it was positive to see some of the mixed groupings from the group work staying together and continuing with the earlier discussions.

Activities

After lunch there was an opportunity to take part in some of the services and activities offered by the hospice, e.g. art therapy, aromatherapy, massage, hand and nail care. The art therapy session was a delightful success as the Art therapy room had been one of the new innovations in Day Therapy's refurbishment. We knew that patients had found it very therapeutic to use art as a means of communication but at the Listening Day patients had an opportunity to draw and paint with their carers. For some it was the first time in a long time that they had been able to do something together that was not related to the illness.

This activity in particular drew our attention to the special needs of carers. The carers who came to the Listening Day were very tired and the opportunity to sit and rest knowing that their loved ones were busy and safe was a treat for some.

The other therapies were a great success also. These therapies were 'a bit of pampering'; a luxury, a treatment which did not involve chemicals or radiotherapy and which emphasised the service users as human beings with worth and dignity.

Throughout the day the service users had been invited to put comments on a paper leaf which was then attached to a 'tree'. This was a great success. The service users were very creative in both their ideas and how they decorated the paper leaves. It also gave anonymity to those who might choose to be less than complimentary. We have found that throughout our service user experience, no matter how many times we emphasise that compliments are all very well and nice but they do not help with service development, we are often ignored and the compliments come anyway.

Altogether the staff and service users felt that the day had been worthwhile and it will be repeated. Lessons have also been learned and some things will be tackled in a different way.

2005–2006

The aims for the Service User Forum for 2005 have been to continue its development. We now employ someone on a part time basis to ensure that the commitment continues and we look forward to seeing how this post develops in 2006. We also intend to involve other service users including bereaved clients, clients out in the community, carers plus more involvement from Bedded Unit patients.

However, much has been achieved as the following list indicates:

- service users, professionals and volunteers are all in agreement that the Service User Forum at Dove House Hospice has been so far a good idea
- we need to employ a member of staff whose specific role is to ensure service user opinions continue to be heard
- a number of service user ideas have been put into action and a further number are awaiting action
- some service user ideas have been rejected – but with explanation
- we need to accept that there are some things we will never get right
- the forum so far has been Day Hospice/Therapy based – it is time to move beyond this and include other service users – but with care
- we have to pay attention to staff issues and opinions on this subject
- we need to do research on the subject and take part in research taking place elsewhere
- we need to get beyond the hospice (if that is what the service users wish) and use our findings in other local and national initiatives
- we need to consider the service users who do not want to attend or are too ill to attend a group meeting
- we need to consider services users who may have a learning disability or a dual diagnosis or do not speak English
- we need to consider standards and audit
- is the Service User Forum time limited? Will the enthusiasm remain when the builders have gone?
- we need to have a Service User Study Day to share our findings with other organisations and to learn from them.

Conclusion

There is no doubt that the service user experience at Dove House Hospice is slowly but very surely changing the culture of how we work. The involvement of service users, in particular patients, in the day to day workings of the hospice is becoming a regular occurrence. Something that once filled us with concern and occasionally anxiety no longer does so. Service user involvement is now part of the fabric of the organisation. It is up to all of us therefore, staff and users, to develop it further and to ensure that complacency does not fill the gap left by our initial concerns.

There is still a long way to go. By and large, service users continue to be very pleased with the services they receive and what concerns they have are not about the specialist palliative care services they receive as a result of their illnesses. Rather their concerns are about peripheral issues that will make their time at the hospice more comfortable.

Acknowledgments

With acknowledgments and thanks to all the Service Users and staff at Dove House Hospice.

Judith Hodgson BA, CQSW, Adv Dip Counselling, PGCE, has been a qualified social worker since 1977 and has had experience of working with service users in the community, in hospitals and for the last fifteen years at Dove House Hospice in Hull. She is currently also seconded to the University of Hull where she has responsibility for the Loss Bereavement and Palliative Care and the Enhancing Communications Modules on the BA Social Work programme.

At Dove House Hospice Judith is the Senior Lecturer in Psychosocial and Education Services and leads teams of social workers, educators and spiritual care workers. Judith is also Vice Chair of the Association of Palliative Care Social Workers and a Trustee of Help the Hospices.

CHAPTER 17

Listen to what we say

Help the Hospices' User Involvement Initiative

Help the Hospices' User Involvement Initiative takes the form of a group of palliative care service users who take the lead in supporting the development of user involvement at national and local level.

Government policy emphasises the importance of public, patient and user involvement in health and social care with patients and service users at the centre of policy and practice. But how do you make that real? And how do you make it work for palliative care service users, a group facing particular difficulties, whose views are particularly at risk of being left out because they may be experiencing pain, serious illness and have limited time and energy?

Key aims of the group are to address issues of diversity and equality as effectively as possible, and demonstrate the contribution that service users can make.

What are key issues for service users in palliative care?

Being told the truth
Some people have the feeling that the person who is ill shouldn't know about their situation. That may be so with some people, but I feel all the people I have met have wanted to know and most knew before the prognosis was given. It is important that precious time is not wasted with irrelevant rules and regulations. Make sure that the necessary services are in place and the family get all the support that is important. This allows the service user with a life-limiting illness to live life up to the hilt, cramming in as much as they can and want to until their day comes.

Being involved
Professionals can read textbooks on the main structure of the illness, but the patient can explain how it affects them. Something that might seem unimportant, like a pillow wedged on one side of the body to protect an area in pain, might not be in a book, but will help when someone comes along with a similar situation. It is easy to exclude the service user when planning their care and support, but it will help if they are included.

I have used both in-patient and out-patient palliative care services provided by my local hospice. The support I received has been helpful but there have been difficulties. The two most difficult areas have been in accessing consistent information and in staff attitudes.

There is a need for change in policy and practice in hospice provision. Because of its roots, hospice care is steeped in a medical model approach to patient care. This makes it hard for people to be treated as whole people. It is all the more vital for the approach to come from a social model perspective as people with life-limiting conditions are usually aware that they have less time and that it must therefore be used to the best advantage. There is an issue around diagnosis and prognosis, and doctors, while able to make some predictions, can get both horribly wrong and so spoil people's 'end of life' experience. However, there is the view, and I hold it, that all of us have a finite time on earth and we should make the best use of it.

How to involve palliative care service users

In order to attract service users to become part of meetings and conferences, and other information-giving and training processes, people need to have a clear idea of why they should become involved and participate, what will be in it for them and how they can contribute to and influence outcomes. They will need to be clear that while their own experiences are valid and useful, they must not dominate. What is required are good listening skills and the ability to use that information to evaluate services provided against standards set down. People with life-limiting conditions will want to know how the hospice movement will meet their needs in relation to becoming part of involvement and participation, and what information and training they will receive in order to do the job.

Including everybody: addressing diversity

There should be no barriers of any kind, no matter who we are or what ails us. We all face the same feelings and suffer equal grief. We can support each other and give each other the will to keep fighting bureaucracy to make life as easy and respectful as possible for everyone.

Men

The main issue I wish to raise about men is that many find it difficult talking in general circumstances about personal issues, and my general experience of cancer patients is that the more forthcoming get more help and that some attention needs to be given to those that find it difficult to cry and express themselves, who hide away feelings and create other problems for themselves.

Black and minority ethnic communities

My story started five years ago, I was given six months to live by my consultant who told me on my discharge from hospital to tidy my affairs up, as I have at most 12 months to live. During my stay in hospital I spoke to a Jewish Rabbi, a couple of Christian ministers, but no Muslim minister, or ethno-sensitive spiritual guidance, or anybody else from a south Asian background, apart from family and friends. Yet some trusts in England have Muslim Imams visiting the wards and employed by the trust. For example, North Birmingham Trust, a trust in Leicester and couple of trusts in London.

The way to engage the black and minority ethnic community, is to sell the idea of hospices, not as a hospital, but as a home from home, where a person can live with dignity. It needs to be offered as an area of respite with all the medical staff around. Diversity is not just a question of colour, whether it is black or white. It is about creating an inclusive society and catering for every interest group and not excluding anyone irrespective. You can't be holistic towards an individual, without being holistic towards their community.

People with different conditions

Hopefully we'll be able to do a lot more to waken people's ideas about what non-malignant diseases (diseases other than cancer) do to people. There's a lot of life-threatening conditions out there, and I want to make sure that hospices and people outside are aware.

My own experience of palliative care has been sparse. As a patient with COPD (chronic obstructive pulmonary disease) I have received little support in palliative care. My social services care is from the care of the elderly and dementia team, so although I am 43 now, I have to pretend that I am in my 80s and suffering short-term memory loss! Well I suppose my body meets the criteria and the high dose of morphine I am on makes me forget things. But seriously in my area, palliative care is only for patients with cancer.

Family and friends

Often they treat you with kid gloves and it's not helpful.

It is always hard for friends and families to come to terms with the fact that someone dear to you is not going to get better. Since becoming ill and my illness reaching 'end stage', has cost me old friends and exclusion from family events, like weddings, christenings and even birthday bashes, because if I am invited my illness gatecrashes. Unfortunately, my illness and I are one person. I can't leave it with a babysitter. I think people are under an illusion that I will burst into tears and discuss what ails me 24/7. How wrong they are! I am probably more likely to be the one cracking jokes (the only problem is that then I end up peeing myself!) – or then I'll probably drop off to sleep given my high level of pain relief. My oxygen can be a pain when someone wants a fag too! But most importantly, I am still me as everyone is themselves, no matter what ails them.

You can't choose your neighbours

When I'm in my own environment I take the opportunity of meeting with people who have similar opinions to me and enjoy the things I enjoy – theatre, music, films and politics. When you go in to hospice, or hospital, you meet with a range of people. When I was in hospital this week, I met someone in the opposite bed who lives near me. He drinks excessively, gambles excessively, has been involved in fighting and is essentially as close to any member of a fascist party I have ever met. It made me think as he loudly expressed his opinions about a range of issues which I totally disagree with. I can't fight with him as a fascist as I would in the old days. Now I let it all go. He was so rude to everyone that it made me realise that we have to cope with this. I can't think where I would normally meet him in the circles I normally move in, and yet he lives two minutes from me. Oh well!

Time is precious for us

Living with a life-limiting illness makes time precious, so making changes in the way patients are treated is important. There are many holes in the care system that need to be filled.

Groups of palliative care service users go down in numbers as well as up

Sadly our groups will decrease as well as increase in size because of the life-limiting nature of people's illnesses, but we should not be excluded just because we are ill. It is very important for us to be heard so that necessary changes can be made in services. It also gives the service user a chance to see improvements being made, thus leaving an important imprint for others to see.

Why we should be involved

There are different degrees of user involvement across hospices nationally at present. No service users are involved in my local hospice. Hospices need to be influenced by patients. They need to take consideration of what patients want. Patients should have a voice in what is being provided for them. There are still issues of stigma for service users with hospices and that's got to change.

People who have life-limiting conditions may not always have the energy or feel well enough to engage in meetings and conferences and other activities, but it must not be assumed that no one can get involved and participate. We are capable of having a view and a knowledge base that is of great value and is there to be tapped into by hospice professional staff. We want to write more than poetry, however important that may be! We can assist with ideas on breaking down barriers between family members, friends and hospice staff, providing creativity in our approaches, if only you will let us truly be an equal and inclusive part of the hospice movement.

Dedication

Karen Willman, a founding member of the Help the Hospices' User Involvement Initiative, died in 2007. She was involved in planning the very first national conference on user involvement in palliative care in 1999 and played a key role in developing user involvement in this field as a service user subsequently, at both national and local levels. She made an enormous contribution to advancing the voice of the service user and this chapter is dedicated to her.

Munir Lalani, service user.
Di Cowdrey, service user.
Mandy Paine, service user.
Karen Willman, service user.
David Hart, service user.
Anne Macfarlane, service user.
Suzy Croft, convener, trustee, Help the Hospices.
Peter Beresford, OBE service user consultant, Centre for Citizen Participation, Brunel University.

References and bibliography

Chapter 8

1 Heron J, Reason P. The Practice of Cooperative Inquiry: research *with* rather than *on* people. In: Reason P, Bradbury H, editors. *Handbook of Action Research*. London: Sage; 2001.

2 Reason P, Bradbury H, editors. *Handbook of Action Research*. London: Sage; 2001.

3 Stock Whitaker, D. *Using Groups to Help People*. Hove: Brunner-Routledge; 2001.

4 Doel M, Sawdon C. *The Essential Groupworker*. London: Jessica Kingsley; 1999.

5 Goldberg S, Muir R, Kerr J, editors. *Attachment Theory*. London: The Analytic Press; 1995.

6 Heegaard M. *When someone special is seriously ill*. London: Jessica Kingsley: 1988.

7 Landry-Dattee N, Delaigue-Cosset MF. Support groups for children. *Eur J Palliative Care*. 2001; 8(3): 107–110.

8 Parkes CM, Relf M, Couldrick A. *Counselling in Terminal Care and Bereavement*. Leicester: British Psychological Society; 1996.

9 Robertson C, Shaw J. *Participatory Video*. London: Routledge; 1997.

Chapter 12

1 Wykurz G, Kelly D. Developing the role of patients as teachers: literature review. *BMJ*. 2002; **325**: 818–21.

2 Department of Health. The expert patient: a new approach to chronic disease management for the 21st century. London: DoH 2001.

3 http://www.dh.gov.uk/Home/fs/en.

4 http://www.nice.org.uk/page.aspx?o=110005.

5 McGuire-Snieckus R, McCabe R, Priebe S. Patient, client or service user? A survey of patient preferences of dress and address of six mental health professions. *Psychiatr Bulletin*. 2003; **27**: 305–8.

6 Fellowes D, Wilkinson S, Moore P. Communication skills training for health care professionals working with cancer patients, their families and/or carers. *The Cochrane Database of Systematic Reviews*. 2004; **2**.

7 Thomson AN. Reliability of consumer assessment of communication skills in a postgraduate family practice examination. *Med Educ*. 1994; **28**: 146–50.

8 Fadden G, Shooter M, Holsgrove G. Involving carers and service users in the training of psychiatrists. *Psychiatr Bulletin*. 2005; **29**: 270–4.

9 Stacy R, Spencer J. Patients as teachers: a qualitative study of patients' views on their role in a community-based undergraduate project. *Medical Education*. 1999; **33**: 688–94.

10 McGarry J, Thom N. How users and carers view their involvement in nurse education. *Nursing Times*. 2004; **100**(18): 36–9.

11 Franks AL. Teaching medical undergraduates basic clinical skills in hospice-is it practical? *Postgrad Med J*. 2000; **76**: 357–60.

12 Baker BL, Joyce JM. Medical student reflects on hospice experience. *J Am Board Fam Practice*. 2003; **16**: 262–4.

13 Cicely Saunders, editor. *St Christopher's in Celebration*. London: Hodder & Stoughton; 1988: p11.

14 http://www.dipex.org/Home.aspx.

15 Dacre J, Richardson J, Noble I, *et al*. Communication skills in postgraduate medicine: the development of a new course. *Postgrad Med J*. 2004; **80**: 711–5.

16 Edmonds P, Burman R, Sinnott C. The goldfish bowl. *Eur J Pall Care*. 2004; **11**(2): 69–71.

17 Todd J. Unpublished data collected from student evaluation and feedback forms after attending a goldfish bowl session at Trinity Hospice, London; 2006.

18 Kennett C, Payne M. Understanding why palliative care patients 'like day care' and 'getting out'. *J Palliat Care*. 2005; **21**(4): 292–8.

19 Wee B, Hillier R, Coles C, *et al*. Palliative care: a suitable setting for undergraduate inter-professional learning. *Palliat Med*. 2001; **15**: 487–92.

20 Cicely Saunders, M Baines, R Dunlop. *Living with Dying*. 3rd ed. Oxford: Oxford University Press; 1995.

Chapter 13

1 Dunker P, Wilson V. *Cancer Through the Eyes of Ten Women*. London: Harper Collins; 1996.

2 McLean G. *Facing Death Conversations with Cancer Patients*. London: Churchill Livingstone; 1993.

3 Lawton J. *The Dying Process: patients' experiences of palliative care*. London, New York: Routledge; 2000.

4 Rogers WA, Draper H. Confidentiality and the ethics of medical ethics. *JME*. 2003: **29**(4); 220–4.

5 Farsides B. Cancer Narratives. *Eur J Cancer Care*. 1999: 8(2); 116–9.

6 Diamond J. *C Because Cowards get Cancer too…*. London: Vermillion; 1998.

7 Picardie R. *Before I say Goodbye*. London: Penguin; 1998.

8 Moran D. *A more difficult exercise*. London: Bloomsbury; 1989.

9 Rose G. *Love's Work*. London: Chatto and Windus; 1995.

10 Conway K. *Ordinary Life: a memoir of illness*. New York: WH Freeman and Company; 1996.

11 Baulby J-D. *The Diving Bell and the Butterfly*. London: Fourth Estate; 1997.

12 Goodare H, editor. *Fighting Spirit: the stories of women in the Bristol breast cancer survey*. London: Scarlet Press; 1996.

13 Arthur I, Arthur T. *Shadow in Tiger Country: one last year of love*. London: Harper Collins; 2000 see also http://www.shadowdiary.com/.

14 Oliviere D, Monroe B, editors. *Patient Participation in Palliative Care: a voice for the voiceless*. Oxford: Oxford University Press; 2003.

15 Medical Humanities databases point one towards a number of plays written about people at the end of life, though the process by which these plays came about would undoubtedly differ from that of *The Tuesday Group*.

16 Clark B. *Whose Life is it Anyway*. London: Samuel French; 1978.

17 Dunn N. *Cancer Tales*. Oxford: Amber Lane Press; 2002.

18 Edson M. *Wit: a play*. New York: Farrar, Straus & Giroux; 1999.

19 Hall L. *Spoonface Steinberg and other plays*. London: BBC Books; 1997.

20 Hawkins AH, Ballard JO, editors. *Time to Go: three plays on death*. Philadelphia: University of Pennsylvania Press; 1995.

Chapter 16

▪ National Institute for Clinical Excellence. *Improving Supportive and Palliative Care for Adults with Cancer.* Guidance on Cancer Services: NHS; 2004.

▪ National Council for Hospice and Specialist Palliative Care Services. *Our Lives Not Our Illness: user involvement in palliative care.* Briefing number 6; November 2000.

▪ The National Council for Palliative Care. *Listening to Users. Helping professionals address user involvement in palliative care.* 2004.